THE REST PRINCIPLE
A Neurophysiological Theory of Behavior

JOHN DAVID SINCLAIR
Research Laboratories of the State Alcohol Monopoly (Alko)
Helsinki, Finland

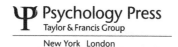

Ψ Psychology Press
Taylor & Francis Group

New York   London

Illustrations in this volume drawn by John David Sinclair

First Published by
Lawrence Erlbaum Associates, Inc., Publishers
365 Broadway
Hillsdale, New Jersey 07642

Transferred to Digital Printing 2009 by Psychology Press
270 Madison Avenue, New York NY 10016
27 Church Road, Hove, East Sussex BN3 2FA

Library of Congress Cataloging in Publication Data
Sinclair, John David.
    The rest principle.

    Bibliography: p.
    Includes index.
    1. Neuropsychology.   2. Neural circuitry—
Adaptation.   3. Reinforcement (Psychology)
4. Psychology—Philosophy.   I. Title.   [DNLM:
1. Neurons—Physiology.   2. Behavior.   WL102.5
S616r]
QP360.S517   612'.8   80-17396
ISBN 0-89859-065-5

Publisher's Note
The publisher has gone to great lengths to ensure the quality
of this reprint but points out that some imperfections in the
original may be apparent.

Contents

Preface

This book represents an attempt to organize nearly the entire field of psychology within a single new theory, based upon only one very simple assumption about neuronal functioning. The gestation period for this theory has been very long. The first parts were developed 15 years ago at the University of Cincinnati, when I was examining some very old ideas, dating back at least to the last century (Wundt, 1874), about optimal levels of stimulation for producing pleasure. Optimal levels of stimulation implied optimal levels of neuronal activity. Because there was an obvious connection between pleasure and reward or reinforcement, this suggested that optimal level of neuronal activity might in some way be related to reinforcement. Reinforcement is anything that increases the probability of a particular pathway of neurons being able to fire again in a similar situation. Therefore, it seemed possible that there might be an optimal level of firing for a neuronal pathway that would cause the connections within this pathway to become stronger. Conversely, levels of firing greatly different from this optimal rate might cause the connections to become weaker.

The idea of an optimal level of firing causing reinforcement was not particularly new. It is likely that much of my thinking at this stage was influenced by William Dember and his hypothesis that an optimal level of complexity was rewarding (Dember, 1965; Dember & Earl, 1957). Although I had little direct contact with him at the University of Cincinnati, his ideas permeated throughout the Psychology Department, and it would have been impossible not to have been influenced by them.

The next step in the development of the present theory took it out of the mainline of psychology and into neurology. I was examining the newly discovered phenomenon that electrical stimulation of certain brain areas produced positive reinforcement (i.e., that rats would bar press for such intracranial stimulation). One possible reason for this appeared to be that stimulation of these particular areas might produce inhibition of the pathways involved in motor acts such as bar pressing. But how could inhibiting a pathway make it become stronger? First, I went back to the idea of the optimal level of firing. If the level of firing were initially too high, inhibition could bring it closer to the optimal level and therefore be reinforcing.

A breakthrough came, however, when I tried viewing this relationship in the opposite way; that is, seeing if reinforcement from inhibition could explain why an optimal level of firing might be rewarding. Suppose connections automatically became stronger in pathways that had just fired when they were allowed or forced not to fire. Suppose, further, that this increase in strength developed more rapidly during the initial part of a rest period. The greatest increase in the strength of connections would then be produced if a pathway fired, then rested long enough for the initial rapid increase in strength, then fired again, then rested for the same duration again, etc. Therefore, there would be an optimal rate of firing for producing the greatest increase in the strength of the connections in the pathway.

The two ideas were thus equivalent, because either one produced the other. The latter idea, which I now call the *rest principle,* was more basic, however, and became the basis for the theory presented in this book. There are actually two sides to this rest principle: First, it states that pathways that rest after firing develop stronger internal connections; and second, it states that pathways that do not rest but go on firing repeatedly develop weaker connections.

During the next five years at the University of Oregon, I found that one after another of the phenomena studied in psychology could be explained by the use of the rest principle. Much of this development occurred in discussions with Joel Adkins, in which we would compare the conclusions obtained with the rest principle with those based upon the alternative *use principle* (i.e., that connections get stronger the more they are used). Needless to say, the rest principle never lost in these comparisons, as is shown in various places throughout this book. There were phenomena that could be modeled equally well with either principle, but there were many cases in which the rest principle produced realistic results, whereas the use principle produced contradictions with known data or conclusions that would probably result in the death of any organism "built" with it.

Also at this time new evidence began to appear suggesting that the nervous system does indeed function according to the rest principle. It has long been known (Peckham & Peckham, 1887) that continued stimulus repetition caused the unconditioned response, such as orienting, to decrease in strength and probability. This is, of course, what the second half of the rest principle says should happen. New evidence now showed that such habituation was a very common, perhaps even universal, phenomenon (Hinde, 1970; Thompsen & Spenser, 1966). In addition to external responses, it was found that habituation occurred in the evoked potential within the brain that a stimulus produces (Cooper, 1971) and in the cortical steady potential response to stimulation (Rowland, 1967). Phenomena like habituation were found in muscles (Katz & Thesleff, 1957; Magavanik & Vyskocil, 1973), sweat glands (Trendelenberg, 1963), the pineal gland (Deguchi & Axelrod, 1973), and in individual neurons (Curtis & Ryall, 1966). So the weakening-of-connections-with-continual-use half of the rest principle appeared to be winning strong physiological support.

The other half of the rest principle also began to win support from new studies on "denervation supersensitivity." It had been known that muscles that have their innervating neurons cut eventually become overly receptive to the transmit-ter substance by which the neurons had previously stimulated them (Langer, 1975). New findings showed that the denervated muscle fibers developed new receptors (Axelsson & Thesleff, 1959), that the muscle was open to innervation by new neurons (Frank, Jansen, Lømo, & Westgaard, 1975), and that similar supersensitivity could be produced merely by inactivating the muscle for long periods of time (Lømo & Rosenthal, 1972). In general, there is a strong similar-ity between the processes involved in neurons stimulating muscle fibers and those involved in neurons stimulating other neurons. Consequently, these find-ings with muscles tended to support the idea that inactivity or rest could produce also an increase in the sensitivity of neurons and thus an increase in the strengths of the inputs into the neuron. This contention has now been verified, because it is now clear that neurons also develop denervation supersensitivity (Costentin, Marcais, Protais, Baudry, DeLaBaume, Martres, & Schwartz, 1977; Crees, Burt, & Snyder, 1977; Feltz & DeChamplain, 1972). It had previously been thought that the development of supersensitivity required several days of inactivity—a time period that was not consistent with the usual time course for learning, but Costentin et al. (1977) have shown that the supersensitivity in neurons is present within 2 hours.

Although the physiological support for the rest principle appears to be grow-ing rapidly, one should not confuse the principle with the possible processes that may underlie it. As shown in this book, the rest principle is thought to be necessary for the development and functioning of nervous systems such as our own. The physiological processes by which the principle is put into action are of secondary importance. Even now the evidence suggests that there is a redun-dancy of processes producing effects in line with the principle. For instance, there probably are both presynaptic and postsynaptic mechanisms for increasing the strength of connections after rest and decreasing it with continual use. The physiological processes are presented in some detail, particularly in Chapter 6, but my interest lies primarily in exploring the implications of the rest principle for mental functioning and behavior.

Aside from a review of the physiological evidence (Sinclair, 1978), I have hitherto been reluctant to publish any of this theory. This is mainly because the evidence for its being the correct explanation for any particular phenomenon is inconclusive: There are undoubtedly other theories that could account also for the phenomenon. Consequently, I do not expect the small amount of evidence pre-sented in this Foreword to convince anyone of the validity of the rest principle. The purpose here has been to give some idea of how the theory developed over the years, not to present it in any logical order—that is what I hope to do in the rest of the book. The strength of the theory lies primarily in the wide range of results that it can explain. Applying the theory to such a wide range of issues has taken a very long time, and it is only now that I am confident enough of the validity of the theory to present it.

Because of the broad general interest in the questions I hoped to address, I started out using a writing style appropriate for Everyman. Unfortunately, he still did not understand completely the first few chapters when he read them, and I saw no hope of being able to present the more technical issues in the later chapters so that he could comprehend, without doing an injustice to the material. Consequently, each section has now been written in the style that seemed to convey most adequately the material in it—and no one will be completely satisfied. The psychologist may be bothered by the oversimplification of the behavioral topics and confused by the technical terms related to physiology, whereas the neurophysiologist may have the opposite reaction: To help lessen these problems, a glossary is included. One bit of advice for the psychologist: Only a few of the neurological and neuropharmacological terms have to be understood in order to follow the discussion (and these generally have been defined in simpler language); the rest can be treated as arbitrary symbols and passed over with relative impunity. For instance, it is of little importance for the arguments whether fluphenazine, alpha-methylparatyrosine, or gobbledygook was used to create supersensitivity; the only important point is that a transmitter has more effect on neurons after the receptors for this transmitter have been forced to rest for a while and that this mechanism is thus able to contribute to rest principle control of neural connections.

It is customary to conclude forewords with acknowledgments to all those individuals who facilitated progress on the work. Out of contrariness, I am tempted to write instead a negative acknowledgment to those who impeded progress. In a way, they too have been helpful, because of my contrariness; perhaps I never would have continued theoretical work if the first professor to whom I gave a theoretical paper had not harshly rejected it because in the assignment he had not asked for a theory.

Nevertheless, I will stick to positive acknowledgments. First there are the individuals whose ideas contributed to the initial development of the theory, particularly Joel Adkins and William Dember. I also want to thank R. J. Senter for his personal encouragement and "patronage" over the years.

The preparation of the book has been made possible by the support and cooperation I have received at Alko, especially from Kalervo Eriksson and Olof Forsander. I wish to thank John Londesborough, John Denslow, Kai Lindros, Dale Bender, Kalervo Kiianmaa, and my other colleagues at Alko for their helpful comments and suggestions and to apologize to them for having diverted every conversation in the last two years around to my theory. I am grateful to the staffs of the departments of psychology of the University of Helsinki and The Center for Advanced Study in Theoretical Psychology, Edmonton, Alberta, for having arranged special series of lectures in which I could present these ideas and for the feedback they provided. Most of all, I wish to thank my wife, Kirsti, for her patience and consideration and for her insight, which has often proved to be quite profound, on many of the issues presented in the book.

1 Introduction

The human brain is the most complex object on Earth that can be studied scientifically: a collection of over 100 billion neurons squeezed into a space about the size of a grapefruit, which somehow is able to control all that you feel, do, and know. We understand rather well how the individual neurons function, how they carry information from one place to another, and how they stimulate or inhibit one another. We even have some idea of how they can analyze the incoming information and how they can organize the production of a response. In between the analyzed stimuli and the response automatons, however, is an area of profound mystery. Although prodigious amounts of data have been collected, there still is little understanding of the most important and interesting functions of the brain, such as what really happens up there when you learn something, when you are thinking, or when you are feeling happy.

This lack of understanding has been caused partly by an antitheoretical attitude in psychology in the last few decades (Royce, 1976). Prior to that, the development of general theories of learning had held an important position in the field. Perhaps because these efforts were not successful, succeeding generations of psychologists came to feel that little was to be gained by trying to make general theories. Instead, they collected information that was, at most, organized into models encompassing only small limited amounts of data. In the process they have made valuable contributions, and our knowledge about behavior has increased tremendously. Meanwhile, however, the fundamental questions have generally been avoided.

For instance, how does reinforcement really work? Perhaps I should define terms here. *Positive reinforcement* is anything that increases the probability of the preceding response's being emitted again in a similar situation. A hungry rat

1

who receives food after pressing a lever is more likely to press the lever again; the food is, therefore, positive reinforcement.

The response was made in the first place because some collection of neurons fired. These neurons formed the connection between the stimuli that were present at that time and the particular response output. It is generally assumed that the response becomes more likely after reinforcement because the synapses in the intervening pathway were strengthened. But how? How can the presence of food in the mouth or in the stomach increase the connectedness of some set of neurons in the brain?

To make matters more complicated, it is now clear that under the right conditions practically anything can be a reinforcer. This finding is primarily what killed many of the older theories of learning. They had postulated that only things that reduced drives were reinforcers. This is certainly true in the case of the rat's learning to run in order to obtain food. The food reduced the hunger drive and therefore (although it was not stated how) managed to reinforce the running. It has since been shown, however, that rats will eat, even when they are not hungry, in order to have access to a wheel in which to run (Premack, 1962). Is there also a drive to run? Animals will also work in order to see things (Butler, 1953, 1958; Butler & Harlow, 1954), to reach a particular level of stimulation (Girdner, 1953; Harwitz, 1956), or to change the level or type of stimulation (Barnes & Kish, 1958; Kish, 1955; Roberts, Marx & Collier, 1958). Eventually the theorists had to postulate curiosity drives, drives for light, sound, and so on, and drives to change the amount of stimulation. The circularity of this argument should be obvious: Reinforcement was anything that reduced drives, and drives were anything that produced reinforcement when they were reduced. So the question of what is reinforcement was more or less put aside, whereas the question of how it really worked to strengthen connections was not usually considered.

Nevertheless, it had become clear that there were very many types of reinforcers. Moreover, each of these could apparently reinforce nearly all responses. In other words, the firing of practically any set of neurons could, under the right conditions, reinforce almost any other set.

The problem of nonspecificity becomes even more apparent in human learning. I just picked two words randomly out of the dictionary: *worm* and *luster*. Having read these, you already have developed some association between them. If you now free-associated to the word worm, the probability that you would say luster has increased. This dictionary has some 100,000 words, so there were about 5 billion pairs of words that could have been selected and that you could have associated. Whatever reinforced your learning of worm–luster,[1] it must have been able to reach all 5 billion of these possible connections.

---

[1]Sorry about the Freudian connotations of this pair of words. They were randomly chosen. If I had rejected them and insisted upon a less embarrassing pair, the selection would no longer have been random.

Previous learning theories generally can be divided into three categories on the basis of how they assume reinforcement strengthens the connections. The first category includes those theories that do not attempt to answer this question. They may specify what constitutes reinforcement (e.g., drive reduction [Hull, 1943], moderate increases in stimulus complexity [Dember & Earl, 1957], or arousal reduction [Berlyne, 1960]), but they do not specify a mechanism by which these factors manage to reach the pathway that has just fired and then strengthen the connections in it.

The second category contains those theories that assume that reinforcement occurs as a result of the activity of some specific mechanism external to the neurons that produced the response. For instance, Olds and Olds (1965) speculated that there was a network of neurons with reinforcing synapses located in the vicinity of all other synapses that could be strengthened. The activation of these reinforcing synapses somehow strengthens the other synapses nearby that had just fired. A similar idea appears in the hypotheses that particular transmitter substances such as norepinephrine or dopamine may cause reinforcement (Rolls, 1975, pp. 73-89). Both of these suggestions have difficulty accounting for the nonspecificity of learning. They would require an input from nearly all units in the brain into this reinforcing network and a *direct* output from it to all synapses that can be strengthened. No known system in the brain has such widespread direct ramifications. The norepinephrine and dopamine synapses, for instance, constitute only a small fraction of the total number of synapses.

The third category of theories includes those that speculate that connections become stronger because of being used. The more a connection is used, the easier it will be to traverse it in the future. This is what I call the *use principle*. It is found in a very wide range of theories (e.g., Guthrie, 1935; Hebb, 1949), but particularly in those proposed by researchers in human verbal learning and classical conditioning (e.g., Konorski, 1967; Pavlov, 1927). These are fields in which the nonspecificity of learning is most obvious and reinforcement is least obvious. As might be expected, theories employing the use principle can easily account for the nonspecificity of learning, but generally have difficulty explaining why positive reinforcement increases and negative reinforcement decreases the probability of the response being emitted again.

The use principle has become very deeply embedded in our thinking. It can also be seen as an implicit assumption in the thinking of some modern neurochemists and neurophysiologists, who often seem to believe that it is proved by behavioral results and that their task is to find the mechanisms causing it (Nathanson & Greengard, 1977). As we shall see in Chapter 6, this must be a most frustrating task for them.

The use principle seems intuitively obvious. If you want to learn a list of words, you say it over and over again, and eventually you know it. Although the introduction of the *law of effect*—that the consequences of an act and not mere repetition of the act determine whether it will be learned—seemed to contradict the use principle, various ways have been found to reconcile the use principle and the law of effect. At present, the use principle is probably accepted by more workers in the field than any other specific mechanism for strengthening neuronal connections.

This acceptance of the use principle has, I feel, been unfortunate, because it almost certainly is wrong.

As pointed out in the next few chapters, the use principle upon close examination produces some impossible conclusions. The physiological evidence also suggests that the use principle is not only wrong but also backward. In other words, synapses that are fired continually not only do not become stronger but actually become weaker.

The theory that I present here does not fall into any of the three categories mentioned. It does specify a process by which connections become stronger. This process does not depend upon any specific set of neurons external to those involved in the pathway to be reinforced but rather, like the use principle, is assumed to be a property of all neurons. Instead of the use principle, however, it is based on its antithesis, which I call the *rest principle*.

The rest principle states that connections within a pathway of neurons become stronger only if the neurons rest after firing and that the connections will get weaker if the neurons are fired repeatedly without rest.

The physiological evidence in favor of the rest principle is already quite strong and growing rapidly, as discussed in Chapter 6. Many of the phenomena that demonstrate the rest principle have been known for a long time and often have been treated as nuisances, perhaps partly because they did not fit in with a conceptualization based upon the use principle. Phenomena illustrating the increase in strength after rest include: (1) postinhibitory sensitization or rebound, in which neurons that have been made to rest by inhibition become easier to fire or spontaneously more active than normal when they are released from inhibition (Kuffler, 1953; Lake & Jordan, 1974); and (2) denervation supersensitivity, in which neurons (and muscles and glands) that have been allowed to rest by removal of input develop more receptors and become easier to fire (Cannon & Rosenblueth, 1949; Costentin *et al.,* 1977; Creese *et al.,* 1977; Feltz & De Champlain, 1972; Sporn, Harden, Wolfe, & Malinoff, 1976; Vetulani, Stawarz, & Sulser, 1976). Phenomena demonstrating the decrease in strength after continual firing include: (1) habituation (Cooper, 1971; Hiude, 1970; Peckham & Peckham, 1887; Thompson & Spenser, 1966); (2) pharmacological desensitization (Changeux, 1975; Curtis & Ryall, 1966; Katz & Thesleff, 1957; Magavanik & Vyskocil, 1973; York, 1970); and (3) denervation subsensitivity (which occurs when the degenerating neuron is flooding the recipient organ with very large amounts of transmitter—the supersensitivity begins developing only after the presynaptic neuron is apparently depleted of transmitter) (Deguchi & Axelrod, 1973; Emmelin, 1964a, 1964b; Reas & Trendelenburg, 1967; Trendelenburg, Maxwell, & Pluchino, 1970). Presynaptic negative feedback, in which the amount of transmitter released is decreased after large amounts have been released and increased if little or no transmitter has been released, appears to contribute both to the weakening of connections with continual use and to their strengthening after rest (Stjärne, 1975).

I remember that many years ago, when I took an introductory course in computer programming, there was one cardinal rule that could not be broken without dire consequences: "Don't program an endless circle into the computer!" If you did, the computer would get stuck until one of its disciples pulled the plug.

The use principle can easily lead to an endless circle, because it involves positive feedback (i.e., the more a system is used, the stronger it gets, thus increasing the probability that it will be used again). The rest principle, on the other hand, involves negative feedback (i.e., systems that are used too much become weaker and therefore are less likely to be used in the future). Consequently, as shown in the next chapter, animals whose nervous systems work according to the use principle are likely to get stuck on one response, but animals whose nervous systems work according to the rest principle do not usually get stuck. I think evolution would have imposed even stronger penalties for endless circles than those we faced in the computer course.

This is only one of the advantages of the rest principle. Another is that it has a built-in process for weakening as well as strengthening connections; in contrast, the use principle allows only increases. This property has made it difficult for theories based on the use principle to deal with punishment and extinction, neither of which presents a problem for the rest principle. Some theorists (Hebb, 1949) have added a *disuse principle* to the use principle (i.e., connections that are not used become weaker). This addition has also produced problems and has not been generally accepted by use principle theorists.

In Chapter 5, it is shown how a nervous system employing the rest principle would automatically develop reciprocal lateral inhibition and self-inhibition, just as it seems our nervous systems do. The combination of the rest principle and these inhibitory connections that would develop from it are then shown to account for a wide variety of the findings presently known to psychology and neurology.

So far I have been emphasizing the differences between the present theory and previous ones. There are also, however, many similarities that should be pointed out.

My idea that reinforcement occurs because pathways that have just been active are allowed or forced to rest is somewhat similar to Guthrie's (1935) "trial terminator" hypothesis: Reinforcement is effective because it changes the stimulus input and thus lessens the chances of interference developing with the response that produced the reinforcement. The major difference is that I postulate an active mechanism for strengthening the last-used pathway during the pause.

Konorski's (1967) proposal for what constitutes reinforcement is also somewhat similar to mine. Like Guthrie, he employs the use principle, but with the modification that associations are formed only when the organism is in a state of arousal. Physiological drives are able to produce this arousal, and therefore all acts produced by a hungry animal, for instance, will be associated with hunger. In order to eliminate unsuccessful responses, Konorski postulates that "retroactive inhibition" rather than interference suppresses the movements that do not interrupt the drive and thus do not reduce the motor arousal. The successful response, however, reduces arousal, is not subjected to retroactive inhibition, and therefore remains strong. Food in the mouth rather than, for instance, an increase in the level of blood glucose is seen as the primary factor for reducing hunger drive.

The present theory, although based on the rest principle, also predicts that arousal is important, although not essential, for the strengthening of connections, as shown in Chapter 10. It is also similar in predicting that stimuli previously associated with the reduction of hunger, such as food in the mouth, are primarily responsible for reinforcing food procurement responses. In this way it resembles also the explanation Rolls (1975) gives for reinforcement from intracranial electrical stimulation. He states that reinforcement is caused by the firing of systems that constitute AND gates for the presence of the physiological need and of stimuli that previously have occurred just before reduction of these needs. Electrical stimulation of these AND gate systems is also reinforcing, and therefore animals will learn to work for such intracranial stimulation. The present theory is in complete agreement with this suggestion and also, I believe, is able to show in a self-consistent manner why it should be so.

The theory therefore is not opposed to most of Hull's drive reduction theory (1943). Indeed it provides a mechanism by which both drive reduction and secondary reinforcement could affect the previously used neuronal pathways and make them stronger.

There is an even closer relationship with those theories suggesting that reinforcement is caused by optimal levels of various factors: optimal levels of receptor stimulation (Leuba, 1955; Wundt, 1874); optimal amounts of stimulus departure from an adaptation level (McClelland, Atkinson, Clark & Lowell, 1953); optimal levels of "perceptualization" (McReynolds, 1956); optimal flow of information from the environment (Glanzer, 1958); optimal levels of stimulus complexity or novelty (Dember & Earl, 1957); and optimal levels of arousal (Berlyne, 1960; Hebb, 1955). As mentioned in the Foreword, the present theory really is an outgrowth of these optimal level theories. It is shown more specifically in Chapter 8 how such optimal levels for reinforcement are a direct corollary of the rest principle. Moreover, because the rest principle is assumed to apply to all neurons, there should be optimal levels of firing at the stimulus input level, at the level of analysis at which neurons are sensitive to stimulus change, and at still higher levels of analysis at which neurons are excited by specific features of the stimuli. It therefore encompasses all the previous optimal level hypotheses. The present theory, however, does not stop there. It also states that there should be optimal levels of firing for the neurons involved in thinking, decision making, response production, and motor control.

I disagree with Berlyne's (1960) conclusion that the reinforcement associated with these optimal levels is caused entirely by arousal reduction. The theory does predict, as mentioned before, that moderate increases in arousal can be reinforc ing in some circumstances. In that sense the theory is in agreement with Berlyne's proposal that the reinforcing properties of, for instance, humor and art may be partially caused by what he calls "arousal jags" (i.e., small brief increases in arousal).

The present theory, with its emphasis on lateral inhibition coming from any strongly activated neuronal pathway, resembles Pavlov's (1927) speculation that excitation of one point on the cortex induces inhibition in the surrounding area, although the inhibition is now seen as being generated by inhibitory interneurons and not by field effects. Nevertheless, many of the conclusions Pavlov reached by reference to inhibitory radiation can also be obtained with the present neuronal lateral inhibition.

Perhaps the greatest similarity is with Hebb's (1949) book *The Organization of Behavior*. This may seem surprising inasmuch as Hebb, of all theorists, gives the most explicit presentation of the use principle, and the use principle and the rest principle are almost exact opposites. As often occurs, in this instance the opposites are more similar to each other than they are to things lying on some other continuum.

Rochester, Holland, Haibt, and Duda (1956) showed with computer simulations that Hebb's cell assemblies would not form in the absence of inhibitory connections. Milner (1957) then suggested that vast amounts of inhibition must be present in the cortex, and Berlyne (1960) pointed out that if such inhibitory connections existed, Hebb's cell assemblies might develop and function as Hebb theorized they would.

A corollary of the rest principle is that lateral inhibitory connections, of the type needed for the development of cell assemblies, would develop automatically in many parts of the nervous system (see Chapters 4 and 9). Thus, the rest principle would create a nervous system in which Hebb's cell assemblies would be likely to form.

Actually Hebb foresaw the rest principle. After discussing Dunlap's finding that deliberate repetition of a response may weaken the response and citing the advantages of spaced over massed trials in classical and instrumental learning, he states: "All these things might suggest that the connections involved in learning are (1) somehow weakened by being activated and need a period of recovery before they can function well a second time; but (2) are strengthened, instead, when the period of recovery has been permitted [p. 225]." Instead of seeing this as the basis for strengthening connections on the neuronal level, Hebb tried to explain it away partially on the basis of the macrobehavior of the "phase sequences": that continued activation somehow would "induce a change of frequency properties in the assembly."

A final similarity with Hebb's work lies in what will not be said here. In other words, many of the conclusions he reached are the same as those produced from the present theory; because he has already presented them, they are not discussed in detail here.

Well, now that I have honored Caesar, let us get on with burying the principle that formed the basis of his theory.

2 Simulations of the *Use Principle* and *Rest Principle* with Neutral Stimuli

It is important to compare some of the logical consequences of the *use* and *rest* principles here, because it is primarily the difference between these principles that separates the present theory from many previous ones. I hope I have made it clear in Chapter 1 that the *use principle* is not a "straw man" that I have constructed.

Let us consider what happens to response probabilities with stimulation that is intrinsically neither rewarding nor punishing, first in a hypothethical organism in which the neural connections between the stimulation and the response operate according to the *use principle* and then in one employing the *rest principle*. In reality, the probability that any response will be emitted is determined not by the absolute strength of that response in the situation but, instead, by its strength in the situation relative to that of other responses. In order to include this notion, it is necessary to have at least two responses. Such a situation has been analyzed with very simple computer simulations—so simple they could be put in a programmable calculator such as a Hewitt–Packard 97.

The simulation could be seen as modeling the behavior of simple neuronal networks. I think it will be easier to understand what is happening, however, if we place the networks inside an animal. There are, of course, no organisms existing that have only two mutually exclusive responses, so I have had to invent the creature shown in Fig. 2.1. This might be considered a primordial version of the "push-me–pull-you" from the children's stories about Doctor Doolittle. Like that animal, our push-me–pull-you can move forward and backward with equal ease. These are its two mutually exclusive responses: going to the left (in the figure, R_l), and going to the right (R_r).

This push-me–pull-you has two sensory receptors: one finger on the left and one on the right. The animal lives on a track with a wall at either end. The receptors fire when the wall is touched; the closer the animal is to the wall, the stronger the stimulation. More specifically, the input to the left receptor, S_l, is 1 unit when the middle of the animal is in position 3 (see Fig. 2.1), 2 units when it is at 2, 3 units at position 1, and 4 units at position 0. The input to the finger on the right, S_r, is 1 unit at position 7, 2 at 8, 3 at 9, and 4 at 10.

The two sensory inputs are both connected to both responses. Thus there are four connections: S_l–R_l, S_l–R_r, S_r–R_l, and S_r–R_r (see Fig. 2.2). All learning occurs by changing the strengths of these S–R connections.

Two simple computer simulation programs have been produced. One simulates such a push-me–pull-you in which reinforcement occurs according to the use principle (i.e., the strength of an S–R connection is increased whenever it is used). For instance, if on a given trial the animal is touching the left wall and receiving S_l, and this input helps to make it move to the left, R_l, then the S_l–R_l connection is strengthened slightly, so that S_l is more likely to be able to produce R_l in the future (.1 arbitrary units were used here as the increments in connection strength).

The second simulation is identical to the first, except that reinforcement occurs according to the rest principle. When an S–R connection is used, its strength is first reduced slightly (by .1 unit). Subsequently, if it is allowed to rest, the strength increases. In the simulation reported here, the strength increased by .1 on each of the next six trials if the connection was not used again. When a

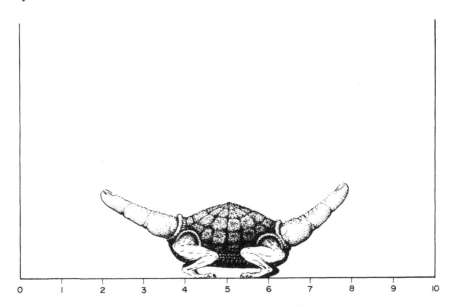

FIG. 2.1.   The primordial push-me-pull-you.

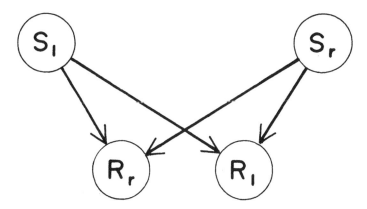

FIG. 2.2.   Connections present in the push-me–pull you. S_l is sensory input from the finger on the left in Fig. 2.1; S_r is sensory input from the finger on the right; R_r is the response of moving to the right; R_l is the response of moving to the left.

connection was used continually, its strength became progressively weaker. For instance, if a connection with a strength of .9 is used for eight trials in a row, its strength would be reduced to .1. If it then is allowed to rest, its strength will return to .7 after six trials but then go no higher.

Initially all connections in both simulations have equal strengths (.5). On every trial the two responses were given a "base strength" between 0 and 1 by a pseudo-random number generator. Stimulus input was then multiplied by the strength of the connections and added to the base strength. For instance, R_r might have a base strength on a particular trial of .673, and R_l of .712, both from the pseudo-random number generator. The animal is in position 1, so S_1 has an input of 3. If the S_l-R_r connection has a strength of .5, then $3 \times .5 = 1.5$ will be added to R_r, giving it a total strength of $1.5 + .673 = 2.173$. If S_l-R_l has a strength of .2, then $3 \times .2 = .6$ will be added to R_l, giving it a total strength of $.6 + .712 = 1.312$. Because R_r is stronger than R_l, R_r will prevail, and the animal will move one position to the right, to position 2.

The usual result from the simulations of push-me–pull-you's with the use principle is shown in Fig. 2.3. If when the animal first touched the left wall, it happened (because of the random base strengths) to continue moving to the left on the next trial, the S_l-R_l connection became stronger. This then made it more likely that it would move even farther to the left. Thus the S_l-R_l connection became progressively stronger until it was impossible for the push-me–pull-you ever to move away from the wall.

If the base strengths for the responses were generated randomly for each individual trial, 75% of the animals ended up immobilized against the walls. Figure 2.4 shows the results of some of these simulations. If the same random

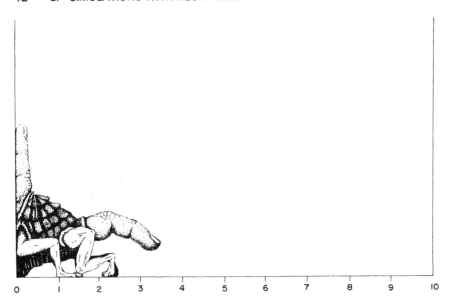

FIG. 2.3.   The usual fate of push-me–pull-you's made with the use principle.

base strengths were used for more than one trial, which may be more realistic than having new ones generated for each trial, an even greater proportion of the use-principle push-me–pull-you's were found to become immobilized against a wall.

Those animals that did manage to avoid immobilization usually had used up all their learning capacity. That is, in these simulations the strengths of the connections were allowed to increased only to 1.0 (i.e., to 100%); the "surviving" animals had the strength of their connections, or at least their S_l–R_r and S_r–R_l connections, increased to 1.0, and therefore no further increases were possible. Consequently, their behavior was essentially random, because it was determined almost entirely by the random base strengths of the responses and not by the stimulus input and the relative strengths of the connections. It had been recognized in the past that a fault of the use principle was that connections could only become stronger, and if there were any maximum strength, it might be reached, rendering the animal incapable of further learning at that location. In order to alleviate this problem, some theorists added the *disuse principle,* as mentioned earlier; That is, connections that are not used become weaker.

Simulations were conducted in which the strength of the connections was controlled both by the use principle and the disuse principle. This did eliminate the problem of the connections making the animals move away from stimulation reaching maximum strength, but it intensified the problem of the animals becoming immobilized against the walls. Given sufficient time, all the animals now became immobilized, with the strength of the connections helping to push them

position

0   10

← trials

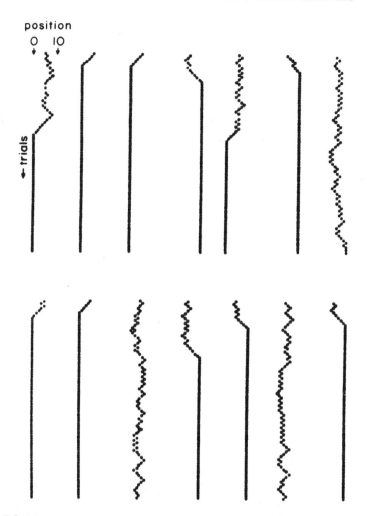

FIG. 2.4.   Results from 80 trials with 14 animals (i.e., 14 different seeds for the random number generater) from computer simulations of the use principle. All but three of the animals became immobilized against one wall or the other.

against one wall reaching 1.0, and the strength of the other three connections falling to 0.

The results with the push-me–pull-you's having the rest principle were quite different. Some of these tests are shown in Fig. 2.5. None of the animals ever became permanently immobilized against the walls. Some wandered back and forth across the track throughout the 80 trials used. Others tended to stay within touching distance of one wall or the other and seldom ventured into the middle area.

position

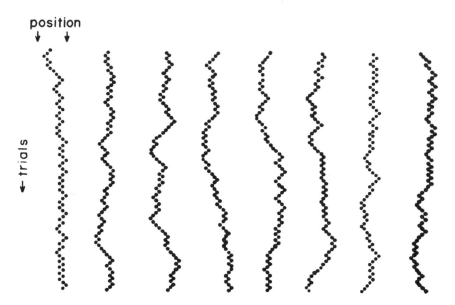

FIG. 2.5.   Results from 80 trials with eight animals from computer simulations of the rest principle. None of the animals became immobilized, and all generally avoided the extreme positions.

In another series of tests, the push-me–pull-you's were driven into one wall by making the base strength of one response much greater than that of the other response. The animals were then allowed to behave "as they wanted" by removing the bias on the base strengths and letting them be determined by the pseudo-random number generator.

The animals with the use principle continued pressing against the wall they had been driven into. The push-me–pull-you's with the rest principle rebounded from the wall as fast as possible and in many cases showed a strong bias against going near that wall again.

The connections in the animals with the rest principle seldom reached full strength, and thus they were seldom without additional learning capacity. If the S_r-R_r or S_l-R_l connections ever reached maximum strength or merely became much stronger than the connections making the animals move away from stimulation, they were quickly reduced by the animal's repeated use of them.

It should be mentioned that this simulation of the rest principle is overly simple. For instance, the strength of the stimulation did not directly affect the changes in the connections: Stronger stimulation merely increased the chances that the response on that particular trial would be determined by the S-R connections rather than by random factors. In Chaper 8, it is shown how the stimulus intensity really does affect the strength of the connections in such a way that animals will be positively reinforced by moderate stimulus intensity and negatively reinforced by strong stimulation. A preview of the latter point can, however, be seen in the present simulations. The prolonged stimulation produced by continually pressing against the wall acted as negative reinforcement. Consequently the animals seldom went all the way to the extreme positions, 0 and 10. Of the 640 trials shown in Fig. 2.5, the animals went to these extreme positions only 36 times. This is less than one-third the number of times that they were in any of the other positions.

It could be argued that this was also an overly simple simulation of the use principle. There certainly are ways in which one could build a push-me–pull-you with the use principle so that it would not spend its life shoving against the wall. For instance, one could put in "pain receptors" that fired when too much pressure was exerted against the finger and then have the firing of these pain receptors somehow disrupt the firing of other pathways. When the animal backed away from the wall and the pain ceased, coherent firing would once again be possible. If we introduce cell assemblies or reverberating circuits into the model, those that were operating when pain ceased would be allowed to continue reverberating and thus would be used more and would become stronger.

This is generally the approach that has been taken by use principle theories. Whenever the use principle by itself produces unrealistic results, new assumptions are added to the theory in order to correct these faults. Thus the theories become more and more complicated. The basic fault of the use principle itself, that it produces "endless circles," is not, however, eliminated. Additional correction mechanisms must then be introduced whenever the theory is applied to new areas.

Incidentally, simplicity has been one of the guiding rules for the development of the present theory. The real reason for this is that I personally get lost when matters become too complicated. I rationalize this by assuming, with some justification I think, that Nature or evolution probably utilized the simplest systems possible in most cases in order to accomplish any function.

Very simple simulations such as those used here are important because they show the basic results produced by the principles themselves, without the addition of corrective mechanisms. I believe these simulations demonstrate that the rest principle produces much more realistic behavior. The results look very much like the behavior we see in animals in the laboratory. It is also the type of behavior that we would expect from people. Imagine that you were in the middle of an absolutely dark room. You probably would walk hesitantly, with your hand extended. When you first touched a wall, you might move a little closer still, perhaps pressing on it a bit. If you were in a brave mood, you might then venture back into the middle and on to the opposite wall. Or you might remain within touching distance of the wall while exploring around the room. I think it is very unlikely you would continue pressing on one spot on the wall for the rest of your life. Moreover, if you happened to rush into a wall, you probably would back away quickly and perhaps have some tendency to avoid going near that wall again.

It should be mentioned that there are creatures such as barnacles and giant clams that do, at one point in their lives, go to a wall and then stay there holding onto it for the rest of their lives. Their behavior is therefore like the use principle push-me–pull-you shown in Fig. 2.3. There also are some psychiatric disorders in which people appear to have "gotten stuck" on one particular response. I cannot comment on the mechanism causing barnacles to "get stuck." The reason some humans get stuck, however, may be related to a useful but potentially dangerous step that may have been taken in evoluation: the construction of special neural junctions, composed of synapses obeying the rest principle but acting as a whole in line with the use principle. As long as these junctions are properly controlled, they improve attention, smooth movements, coping with emergencies, and various other functions, but if for some reason they get slightly out of control, the person is liable to "get stuck" on repetitive response cycles or obsessive thought patterns. This hypothesis is discussed in Chapter 10.

3 Learning to Eat

In Chapter 2 we dealt with a more or less neutral stimulus: touching a wall. We now compare the two principles with a stimulus and response essential for life: hunger and eating. For the sake of visualizing, we again use the push-me–pull-you's. It is assumed that both types of primordial push-me–pull-you's somehow lived through their experiences with the walls and now have developed a mouth, a stomach, and a receptor that signals hunger, S_h (see Fig. 3.1). They have two responses they can make with food: spitting it out, R_{out}, or swallowing it, R_{in}. The hunger receptor is innately connected to both responses, with the initial strengths of the two connections, S_h-R_{out} and S_h-R_{in}, being equal. The animal then has to learn to make the appropriate response.

The situation is therefore somewhat similar to that faced in Chapter 2 because there is one response that removes the stimulation and one that does not. We first consider what would happen if the animals lived in an unrealistically benevolent world in which food were continually falling into their mouths. Some of the conclusions will have to be altered when we later consider a more realistic world in which food is often not present, but the unrealistic situation will serve as a good introduction.

We examine the push-me–pull-you with the rest principle first. We assume that the animals are initially hungry. When food first enters their mouths, by chance half of them will swallow it and half of them will spit it out. Those that swallow it will have their hunger turned off. Consequently, their S_h-R_{in} connection will be allowed to rest until the food is digested and hunger eventually develops again. In the meantime, S_h-R_{in} grows in strength. When hunger does develop again, it is very likely that food will be swallowed, and S_h-R_{in} will be

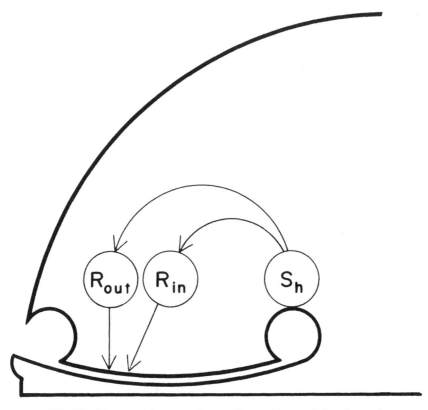

FIG. 3.1.   Diagram of the new push-me–pull-you with a mouth (opening on the
left), throat, and stomach, a receptor (S_h) signaling hunger, and two possible
responses: spitting out the food (R_{out}) and swallowing it (R_{in}). The connections
from the hunger receptor are assumed to be initially equal, and the animal must
learn which response to make on the basis of experience.

further strengthened during the subsequent period of satiation. Thus this half of
the animals will have learned to eat when they are hungry.

The worst that can happen to the remaining half of the animals is that S_h–R_{in}
and S_h–R_{out} will be strengthened equally. If after spitting the food out on the first
trial, they swallow it on the second trial, both connections will be strengthened
optimally during the satiation period, because both fired once and then were
allowed to rest. During the next period of hunger, half of these animals will
swallow the food as their first response and therefore will be likely to learn to
swallow food always when they are hungry. Thus, the proportion of animals
having learned to make R_{in} will be approximately $1 - (.5)^t$ where t is the
number of times that hunger has been present, (i.e., 50% the first time, 75% by

the end of the second hunger period, 87%, 94%, 97%, 98%, 99%, etc.). The actual learning rate might vary from this slightly because of the relative sizes of the increases in strength produced during rest versus the range of variation caused by random effects.

Another factor that would affect the learning rate is the number of trials during which the same random biases on the base strengths of the two responses are present. The preceding figures are found if the biases are generated anew for each trial. If they persisted for more than one trial, the number of animals learning to swallow when hungry would be substantially increased. For that half of the animals in which R_{in} was made on the first trial, such persistent biases would make no difference, because their hunger is gone after the first trial, and their S_h-R_{in} connection would increase as before. The other half of the animals that spit out the food initially would be likely to continue spitting it out for as long as the bias persisted, thus decreasing the strength of the S_h-R_{out} connection through continued use. When the animal finally swallows the food to terminate the hunger period, S_h-R_{in} will receive the full increment added to its strength during the satiation period, whereas S_h-R_{out} will have this increment added to its already reduced strength. Consequently, in the next hunger period S_h-R_{in} will be stronger than S_h-R_{out}, and most of these animals will swallow on the first trial and then proceed to learn the response completely through succeeding reinforcements. Computer simulaions have been conducted and have verified these ideas.

Reinforcement with the use principle, unlike that with the rest principle, is not directly altered by a period when the hunger stimulus is removed. Instead, it occurs whenever a connection is used. If the randomly determined base strengths of R_{in} and R_{out} change with each trial, on the average 50% of the animals eventually will learn always to swallow food when they are hungry, whereas the other 50% will learn to spit it out consistently. If a run of several R_{in} responses occurs randomly before a run of R_{out} responses, the animal will learn to swallow, but if the run of R_{out} responses occurs first, it will learn to spit out the food.

With the rest principle, it was shown that the speed of learning to swallow when hungry was accelerated if the random biases persisted for more than one trial. It might be pointed out that this is probably true in reality. Of the various external factors that might exist for biasing one response over another, it seems likely that some of them would be present for longer than the time between two responses being emitted.

If such long-term biases were present in the animals with the use principle, even less than 50% of them would learn to swallow food when they were hungry. Suppose, for instance, that the biases persisted for the duration of two trials. If swallowing occurred, only one increment in S_h-R_{in} would be produced, because during the second trial, when swallowing again has the stronger base strength, hunger has been removed, and therefore S_h-R_{in} cannot be incremented a second time. If, however, spitting out occurred on the first trial, hunger is not removed,

Therefore, a second trial with S_h firing will follow. The persisting bias will ensure that R_{out} is also emitted on the second trial. Consequently, two decrements in S_h-R_{out} will be produced. Computer simulations of this condition have shown, as would be expected, that approximately twice as many animals learn to spit out the food as learn to swallow it. Random biases persisting for more than two trials result in even larger proportions of the animals learning to spit out food when they are hungry.

Animals with the rest principle would not continue eating once they were full if they had, for instance, a receptor for stomach extension. The output from this receptor alone, however, would not be effective in terminating eating or making an animal spit out food. As discussed in Chapter 9, this requires AND gate neurons that fire only to the combination of stomach extension plus the taste or feel of food in the mouth. The AND gate terminators for eating and drinking develop automatically with the rest principle, but the mechanisms involved will have to be discussed first before this topic can be treated properly.

With the use principle, half of the animals would learn to swallow food when they were full, if the biases on the response-base strengths change with each trial. If the biases persist for more than one trial, more than half would learn to eat in response to not being hungry.

In Chapter 2, it was found that under the best conditions only one-quarter of the use principle push-me–pull-you's did not become immobilized against the walls. We now have lost at least three-quarters of the survivors through their failing to swallow food when they were hungry or exploding when they continued eating after they were full. The same problems would be encountered with thirst and with breathing, so we would be left with only one out of every 256 animals. Clearly, the use principle is not very conducive to survival. The reason is, of course, that survival is dependent upon the keeping of factors within certain limits. This requires negative-feedback homeostatic systems. Such negative feedback is automatic with the rest principle alone, but does not occur with the use principle alone.

It might be argued that all these homeostatic systems are built-in to the animal and do not need to develop with experience. The need for negative feedback, however, does not occur only with the intake of essential substances, but rather is needed for practically all activities (e.g., motor movements, hormonal regulation, and sensory input modulation). It is possible to continue postulating built-in controls on the use principle, such as the specific pain mechanisms to disrupt firing mentioned in Chapter 2, to prevent animals from spending their lives pressing against walls or walking into flames. This eventually would require the postulation of control systems for practically every possible response.

Disruptive pain is clearly not the corrective mechanism for all responses. For instance, look at the X below as long as you can:

X

Why did you stop? If you were built with the use principle, you probably would still be staring at the X.

During the first few minutes that you looked at the X, the stimulation from seeing the X repeatedly preceded the continued emitting of the response of looking at it. These same pathways were used over and over again and therefore should have become stronger and stronger the longer you looked at the X. Unless some particularly strong stimulus intervened at the beginning, you would have continued staring until pain, from starvation perhaps, developed to disrupt what would have been one of your strongest $S-R$ pathways.

It might be argued that the stimulation from the X became weaker, and therefore the response finally stopped. But this would be habituation, the weakening of connections with continual use, and thus opposite to the use principle. So if this argument is made, it is already accepted that at least part of the nervous system, the sensory system, does not work according to the use principle. I could then ask you to think of the syllable *ex* for as long as possible, and when you stopped (before starvation developed), you would have to discard the use principle for the central neurons involved with thinking, too.

Maybe this has been stated too strongly. It certainly is possible to think of a built-in corrective mechanism for the reason you stopped looking at the X that does not undermine the use principle itself. For instance, Hebb (1949) invoked disruptive changes in timing of firing for this purpose. The point is that the use principle requires a huge number of built-in mechanisms to make it function at all realistically. There must first be built-in systems for regulating the intake of food, water, oxygen, and salt. I have shown previously that alcohol drinking by rats seems to be under homeostatic control (Sinclair, Walker, & Jordan, 1973). Is there a built-in corrective mechanism for alcohol drinking? And are there built-in corrective mechanisms for saccharin, quinine, and citric acid intakes that also increase after deprivation (Wayner, Greenberg, Tartaglione, Nolley, Fraley, & Cott, 1972)? Compensatory behavior can also be seen in sexual activity (Beach & Jordan, 1956), socializing (Sloan & Latane, 1974), wheel running (Hill, 1956), and spontaneous alternation (Dember & Fowler, 1958). Are all of these genetically controlled, too? Then there must be other built-in corrective mechanisms for keeping animals from going to very strong stimulation. Then another mechanism must be present to disrupt activities that persist too long. The list could go on and on.

Although it is possible that all these mechanisms might be built into animals, let us proceed with showing how realistic behavior would develop automatically in animals with the rest principle.

The results in this chapter so far have been similar to those in Chapter 2. The animals with the rest principle have learned to swallow food when they are hungry in much the same way that they learned to move away from prolonged contact with the wall. The discussion now becomes a bit more complicated, as we consider what happens to stimuli that accompany the presence of food. This brings us in Chapter 4 to how classical conditioning could work in animals, employing the rest principle.

First, let us give the push-me–pull-you a receptor that reports when food is in the mouth, S_{food}. In order for the animal to know when it is both hungry and food is in its mouth, let us give it a neuron (or collection of neurons) that receives input from both S_h and S_{food}. This unit, S_{h+food}, acts primarily as an AND gate, firing usually only when the combination of both hunger and food in the mouth are present. It is, therefore, a type of sensory unit, or feature detector, that signals the occurrence of a rather specific event.

We will assume that all the sensory units, S_{food}, S_h, and S_{h+food}, have connections with both the swallowing and spitting out responses, and that these connections are initially equal in strength (see Fig. 3.2).

In the first half of this chapter it is assumed for simplicity that food was constantly being put into the animal's mouth. Therefore, the swallowing and spitting out responses could occur only when food was present. The situation is now a bit more realistic in that there are periods when no food is given.

On an intuitive level, it can be seen that S_{h+food} should become strongly connected with R_{in} if the rest principle is employed, just as S_h became connected to R_{in} in the previous rest principle simulation. In that simulation, swallowing

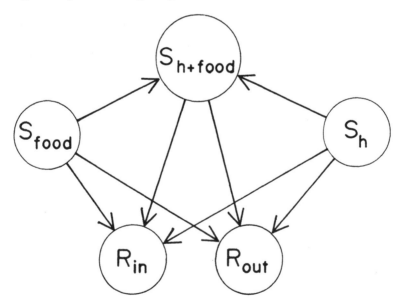

FIG. 3.2. Assumed connections between receptors signaling food in the mouth (S_{food}), hunger (S_h), and the combined presence of both (S_{h+food}), and the responses of swallowing (R_{in}) and spitting out (R_{out}).

invariably eliminated S_h and allowed rest. Now swallowing when *both* food and hunger are present always eliminates S_h and therefore also S_{h+food}. S_{h+food} then rests, and $S_{h+food}-R_{in}$ becomes stronger.

When food is no longer continually present, the dominance of S_h-R_{in} over S_h-R_{out} is reduced. As in the previous simulation, the firing of S_h-R_{in} assures its own rest and consequently will grow stronger. This occurs, however, only when food is present. When food is not present, S_h-R_{in}, being the preferred response, will be used repeatedly until it is weakened to a strength within the range of S_h-R_{out}.

The validity of these conclusions has been tested with two different sets of computer simulations instead of with just one, as had been done previously. The reason for this is that the rest principle deliberately has been left vague as to specific neuronal locations. Most important, it has not been stated whether it is the presynaptic or postsynaptic neuron that must rest in order for the synapse to become stronger. Consequently, one simulation was performed in which postsynaptic rest produced the increase in synaptic strength, and a second in which presynaptic rest was necessary. In both simulations, the presence of food was randomly determined. With the postsynaptic rest model, synapses that were active and contributed to the firing of the postsynaptic neuron became stronger whenever the postsynaptic neuron subsequently rested, the amount of increase in strength being larger on the trials immediately following and going to zero after ten trials had elapsed. When the postsynaptic neuron was active on two trials in a row, those synapses contributing to its activation on the second trial were weakened.

In the presynaptic rest model, on every trial the strength of active synapses was decreased by the value $m^2 e^{-m}$, whereas the strength of inactive synapses was increased by $m^2 e^{-m}$ The only effect of postsynaptic firing was to increase the magnitude of these changes, by setting m back to 1 whenever it fires and having m increase by 1 on each trial in which it does not fire. The formula $m^2 e^{-m}$ is arbitrary and was chosen only because it is maximal when $m = 2$ and rapidly gets smaller as m increases above 2.

The results with both models are shown in Table 3.1.

TABLE 3.1.
Mean Changes in Synaptic Strength after 40 Trials in 15 Animals*.
From Computer Simulations of Two Rest Principle Models

Presynaptic unit	S_{h+food}		S_{food}		S_h	
Postsynaptic unit	R_{in}	R_{out}	R_{in}	R_{out}	R_{in}	R_{out}
Postsynaptic rest model	7.55	2.37	5.30	5.66	4.47	5.87
p that $R_{in} = R_{out}$	.000003		.33		.013	
Presynaptic rest model	8.07	5.79	1.54	0.59	−0.11	−1.28
p that $R_{in} = R_{out}$	.000013		.23		.00087	

*15 different initial seed numbers for the randomizer.

With both models, swallowing became the preferred response when both food and hunger were present (i.e., $S_{h+\text{food}}-R_{\text{in}}$ became much stronger than $S_{h+\text{food}}-R_{\text{out}}$). In both cases only one animal out of 15 failed to learn this in the first 40 trials, and these learned it when an additional 40 trials were given. (In 40 trials, an animal encountered the combination of food and hunger only about six times).

S_{food} did not become preferentially attached to either response in both models. The postsynaptic rest model produced a tendency for S_h to become preferentially connected to R_{out}, whereas the presynaptic rest model produced a more consistent tendency for it to become more strongly attached to R_{in}. Neither tendency was of a large magnitude, and they had little effect on behavior when food was present.

The changes in the connections from S_{food} and S_h to $S_{h+\text{food}}$ were not included in the postsynaptic rest model, because it was obvious that they would both grow rapidly once R_{in} became the preferred response to $S_{h+\text{food}}$. $S_{h+\text{food}}$ must rest whenever R_{in} follows its firing and S_h is removed. The inputs that initially made it fire, that is, the inputs from S_{food} and S_h, will then grow stronger. These connections, however, were included in the presynaptic rest model simulation. The $S_{\text{food}}-S_{h+\text{food}}$ connection did not change significantly, whereas the $S_h-S_{h+\text{food}}$ connection increased significantly.

The absolute size of the changes shown in Table 3.1 are not important because they are determined by the arbitrarily chosen parameters included in the simulations; only the relative changes have importance for the behavior. Nevertheless, it is interesting to note that in the presynaptic rest model, the $S_{h+\text{food}}-R_{\text{out}}$ connection grew in strength, although not so much as the $S_{h+\text{food}}-R_{\text{in}}$ connection. The reason for this is that once the animal had learned always to swallow when both hunger and food were present, the $S_{h+\text{food}}$ inputs to both responses could be present for only one trial before being turned off. The input to R_{out} would not have grown if a slightly more complicated model had been used in which only those synapses that contributed to the initial firing of the postsynaptic neuron could become stronger when they subsequently rested.

There are really a very large number of different models that could embody the rest principle; 320 can be derived from Table 3.2. The postsynaptic rest model simulated here is really model C, b, II, iii, according to the designation in Table 3.2, because the increase in synaptic strength occurred when both presynaptic and postsynaptic neurons fired (C in Table 3.2), and then the postsynaptic neuron rested (b in Table 3.2). Decreases occurred when the postsynaptic neuron fired first (II), and then both the presynaptic and postsynaptic neurons fired (iii). The presynaptic rest model simulated in this example is model B, a, II, i. The model suggested in the preceding paragraph for keeping $S_{h+\text{food}}-R_{\text{out}}$ from increasing in strength would be model C, a, II, i.

The number of rest principle models is further increased if interactions are specified. For instance, a model might state that increases in synaptic strength occur when the presynaptic neuron rests after it fires or when the postsynaptic

TABLE 3.2.
Rest Principle Models

Specific models are produced by choosing one alternative from each of the following sets:

What must fire initially if synaptic strength is to increase subsequently:
  A. presynaptic neuron (= pre)
  B. postsynaptic neuron (= post)
  C. both pre and post
  D. either pre or post
What must subsequently rest if synaptic strength is to increase:
  a. pre
  b. post
  c. both pre and post
  d. either pre or post
What must fire initially if synaptic strength is to decrease subsequently:
  I. pre
  II. post
  III. both pre and post
  IV. either pre or post
  V. neither must fire, but either may fire
What must then fire if synaptic strength is to decrease:
  i. pre
  ii. post
  iii. both pre and post
  iv. either pre or post

---

neuron rests after it fires but not when the presynaptic one rests after the postsynaptic one fires or vice versa.

There is at present little evidence for deciding which of the models is most likely to be correct. Physiological data suggest that there are processes resembling the rest principle occurring in both the presynaptic nerve ending and in the postsynaptic receptor region. Therefore, more general models, such as a D, d, IV, iv model, may be closer to reality. As shown in the present simulations of learning to eat when food was present, it was not necessary to use such general models with the rest principle operating both presynaptically and postsynaptically. The animals learned to eat properly with both of the restrictive models simulated. More general models in which both presynaptic and postsynaptic rest could contribute to increases in synaptic strength would, of course, be expected to be even more efficient in causing the animal to learn to swallow when food and hunger were present.

It should be pointed out that there are also a large number of models for the use principle. Connections could be seen as becoming stronger when only the presynaptic neuron is used, whenever the postsynaptic neuron fires, whenever either is used, whenever both are used, or whenever any of the foregoing is used repeatedly. This raises questions such as whether inhibitory synapses would grow stronger when they are used repeatedly, inasmuch as the presynaptic

TABLE 3.3.

Mean Changes in Synaptic Strength after 40 Trials in 10 Animals from Computer Simulations of the Presynaptic Rest Model in which R_{out} Removes S_{food} for One Trial and R_{in} Removes it for One to Four Trials

Presynaptic unit	S_{h+food}		S_{food}			S_h		
Postsynaptic unit	R_{in}	R_{out}	R_{in}	R_{out}	S_{h+food}	R_{in}	R_{out}	S_{h+food}
	9.45	6.78	7.06	4.52	5.20	1.32	0.36	2.76
$p\ R_{in} = R_{out}$	.000028		.0000002			.0062		

neuron would be firing continually, but the postsynaptic unit would be forced to be silent. Such questions generally have not been faced by use principle theories.

One additional simulation was made of learning to eat when food is present, employing the rest principle. It was the same as the presynaptic rest model simulation, except that the presence of food was no longer completely random. In the real world, either swallowing or spitting out food removes it from the mouth. When it has been spit out, it is still present in the environment and may be taken into the mouth again. If it has been swallowed, it is possible that the animal has exhausted this food supply and will not run into another supply for a while. Consequently, in this simulation, R_{out} eliminated S_{food} for one trial, whereas R_{in} eliminated S_{food} for one to four trials.

The results with this simulation are shown in Table 3.3. As before, S_{h+food} became preferentially connected to R_{in}. This occurred much more rapidly than with the first two simulations: None of the animals spit out food when it was hungry after the fourth trial. This was partly because S_{food} also became preferentially connected to R_{in} and, to a lesser extent, so did S_h. The connections from both S_{food} and S_h to S_{h+food} increased significantly.

This chapter and Chapter 2 have been concerned with showing some of the general consequences of the rest principle. In Chapter 4 we leave the development of the theory for a while and show some of the applications to classical conditioning (e.g., how ringing a bell whenever food is presented eventually causes the bell alone to elicit salivation).

It was important to consider these general consequences for two reasons: (1) in order to give an overview of how the rest principle could make an animal behave; and (2) because these general predictions are at least as important as the more specific predictions about the outcome of controlled experiments. A theory should be able to account for the basic and obvious features of behavior, such as its general flexibility and its homeostatic control. If it cannot explain these features, it is of little importance whether it can account for specific results observed in the laboratory.

Nevertheless, it is also necessary that a theory be in agreement with the specific and sometimes counterintuitive findings from controlled experimentation. So let us take a look at classical conditioning and the rest principle.

4 Classical Conditioning

In Chapter 3, nothing is assumed to be built into the animals' nervous systems that makes S_{food} become able to trigger swallowing in hungry animals. The connections becomes stronger because of an outside contingency: that swallowing when food is in the mouth could remove the hunger stimulation. Consequently, any other stimulus, such as the ringing of a bell, that was invariably present before R_{in} relieved hunger but not present at other times would be expected to develop its own strong connections with R_{in}. This alone could cause classical conditioning to occur. Other factors, however, are at least equally important. There now is an existing strongly connected pathway, S_{food}-(and S_h-) $S_{h+\text{food}}$-R_{in}, that will influence learning. In addition to this pathway itself, it is very likely that there are strong inhibitory connections from the pathway that will also enhance learning.

Let us assume that there is a receptor that is sensitive to the stimulation from the bell (S_{bell}) and also some unit ($S_{h+\text{bell}}$) that receives inputs from S_{bell} and from S_h and fires only when the animal is hungry and the bell rings. Before conditioning it can be assumed that both S_{bell} and $S_{h+\text{bell}}$ have weak connections with all other units, including those in the S_{food}-(and S_h-)$S_{h+\text{food}}$-R_{in} pathway. It is very likely, according to the rest principle, that the latter connections will grow rapidly. For each of these connections, S_{bell}-S_{food}, S_{bell}-$S_{h+\text{food}}$, S_{bell}-S_h, S_{bell}-R_{in}, $S_{h+\text{bell}}$-S_{food}, $S_{h+\text{bell}}$-$S_{h+\text{food}}$, $S_{h+\text{bell}}$-S_h, and $S_{h+\text{bell}}$-R_{in}, the presynaptic neuron fires when the bell is rung (assuming the animal is hungry during training). The postsynaptic neuron in each case is then fired when the food is presented. Subsequently, it is likely that all these units, both presynaptic and postsynaptic, will rest and cause the connections to grow. Hunger is removed, so $S_{h+\text{bell}}$, S_h, and $S_{h+\text{food}}$ will rest. If another trial is not given immediately,

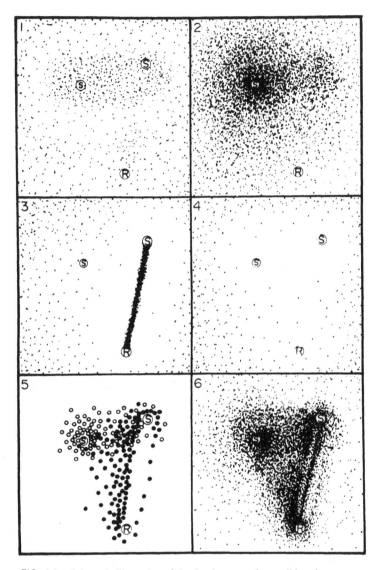

FIG. 4.1.   Schematic illustration of the development of a conditioned response,
such as salivation in response to a bell, after it has been followed by giving food to
the hungry animal. The dots represent neurons firing. The small *s* on the left of
each frame represents a neuron or set of neurons fired only by the combination of
the conditioned stimulus, CS, (e.g., the bell) and the preexisting state (e.g.,
hunger, or, in another conditioning paradigm, the expectation of an air puff to the
eye). The larger *S* on the right is a unit or units fired by a combination of the
preexisting state and the unconditioned stimulus, UCS, (e.g., hunger and food). *R*
is the unconditioned response, UCR, (e.g., salivation and eating). In frame 1 only
the preexisting state is present. In frame 2, the CS is present, and a large number of

both S_{bell} and S_{food} probably will not fire and, in the absence of S_{food} and S_{h+food}, R_{in} is unlikely to fire again.

The resting of the presynaptic units, S_{bell} and S_{h+bell}, and of intermediate neurons triggered by them, is further assured by lateral inhibition (i.e., the strong inhibitory connections that a frequently used pathway develops onto other pathways). How the rest principle causes these lateral inhibitory connections to develop is shown in Chapter 5. The inhibition from the pathways involving eating perhaps may be seen in the suppression of other behavior and the difficulty in disrupting eating by other stimuli. During the rest caused by the inhibition from the firing of the S_{food}-(and S_h-)S_{h+food}-R_{in} pathway, connections that have just been fired, such as those from S_{bell} and S_{h+bell}, will grow stronger.

Lateral inhibition has been found in various systems to decrease with distance from the source, and it is reasonable to assume that it does so elsewhere in the brain. This characteristic also helps assure that the bell will elicit R_{in}, as summarized in Fig. 4.1. This figure shows specifically how an S_{h+bell} unit or units would become strongly connected to R_{in}. The black dots illustrate firing neurons, the s represents S_{h+bell} for the present example, S represents one or more S_{h+food} neurons, and R represents R_{in}.

In frame 1, before the bell is rung, only S_h is present, and neurons with input from it, located in the upper half of the frame in the region of s and S, are firing more rapidly than are neurons elsewhere. In the second frame, the bell is ringing and S_{h+bell} is firing and eliciting firing from a large number of other neurons: The number of excited neurons is assumed to decrease as a function of the distance from s. In frame 3, the bell has stopped ringing, and food has been given, causing S (i.e., S_{h+food}) and the pathway to R (i.e., R_{in}) to fire. Because this pathway is strongly developed and produces lateral inhibition, the firing of neurons elsewhere is reduced. The inhibition is strongest near the pathway, and the firing of other neurons here is completely suppressed. Neurons just fired by S_{h+bell} that are close to the pathway will be forced to rest and therefore will develop stronger synapses, so that in the future they will be excited more easily

---

neurons triggered indirectly by it are firing. In frame 3, the UCS is present and triggering the UCR via a strongly connected pathway and, in the process, suppressing firing of other neurons by lateral inhibition from the UCS–UCR pathway. In frame 4, the preexisting state has been removed, and neurons previously excited by it are resting. Frame 5 shows regions of CS-triggered units whose synapses have been strengthened primarily by inhibition from the UCS–UCR pathway (●), or primarily by removal of the preexisting state (○). Notice that the ● units are most concentrated in the region bordering the UCS–UCR pathway, where inhibition is strongest, and therefore are the CS-triggered units most likely to excite this pathway are R_{in}. There also are more ● units near s, since the increase in synaptic strength is dependent on their having been fired initially, as well as subsequently being inhibited. In frame 6, the CS is presented again, now more easily triggers those units whose synapses have been strengthened, and therefore is more likely to elicit R.

by $S_{h+\text{bell}}$ and will be more able to fire additional units. Because they lie next to $S_{h+\text{food}}$ and R_{in} and the pathway between them, it is likely that they have synapses on them and will be able to elicit R_{in}. Neurons triggered by $S_{h+\text{bell}}$ but lying far away from the $S_{h+\text{food}}$–R_{in} pathway will experience less inhibition and may continue firing. Their synapses will therefore be weaker than those of the units near the pathway.

In frame 4, food has been swallowed and hunger eliminated. Firing in the region stimulated by S_h is thus reduced (and also probably actively inhibited by features not shown here). Consequently, $S_{h+\text{bell}}$ and $S_{h+\text{food}}$ and the neurons excited by them will be allowed to rest and their synapses to grow. This will particularly increase the likelihood that $S_{h+\text{bell}}$ will be able to fire $S_{h+\text{food}}$, but it will also tend to strengthen the connections from the $S_{h+\text{bell}}$-triggered unit to the $S_{h+\text{food}}$–R_{in} pathway and to R_{in} itself, because the inputs from both $S_{h+\text{bell}}$ and $S_{h+\text{food}}$ have been eliminated.

Frame 5 shows the regions of neurons excited by $S_{h+\text{bell}}$ that have their synapses strengthened primarily by inhibition from the $S_{h+\text{food}}$–R_{in} pathway (●) and those strengthened primarily by removal of S_h (○).

Frame 6 shows the next trial after S_h has returned, when $S_{h+\text{bell}}$ is fired again. Neurons in the direction of the $S_{h+\text{food}}$–R_{in} pathway now have stronger connections from $S_{h+\text{bell}}$ and probably stronger synapses onto the pathway. Therefore, they are more likely to be fired now and in turn to trigger the $S_{h+\text{food}}$–R_{in} pathway and R_{in}.

It should be pointed out that Fig. 4.1 is still an oversimplification. $S_{h+\text{bell}}$, $S_{h+\text{food}}$, and R_{in} units would probably be found in a multitude of locations. Nevertheless, the conclusions from Fig. 4.1 would still be true: The closer neurons fired by $S_{h+\text{bell}}$ units are to $S_{h+\text{food}}$–R_{in} pathways, the more likely they are to be inhibited by these pathways when food is given and therefore to rest and develop stronger synapses.

In summary, the conditioned response would develop because of: (1) inhibition from the $S_{h+\text{food}}$–R_{in} pathway; and perhaps also from the S_{food}–$S_{h+\text{food}}$ and S_{food}–R_{in} pathways; (2) removal of S_h; and (3) if increases in synaptic strength either depend upon or are enhanced by postsynaptic rest, also by the fact that the neurons in the S_{food}–(and S_h–)$S_{h+\text{food}}$–R_{in} pathway are assured of being fired and then resting.

In contrast with our analysis in previous chapters with push-me–pull-you's, the present analysis of the development of a conditioned response has been seen as involving a large number of interneurons: facilitory interneurons lying between $S_{h+\text{bell}}$ and the $S_{h+\text{food}}$–R_{in} pathway and within the later pathway, as well as inhibitory interneurons from the pathway. The use of polysynaptic connections lessens the differences between the many different rest principle models. For instance, in the pathway A–B–C–D: If B and C both fire and then rest, the pathway gets stronger, regardless of what model is used. If the presynaptic neuron must fire and then rest for increases in synaptic strength to occur, the synapses between B and C and between C and D will get stronger. If the postsynaptic neuron must fire and then rest, the connections between A and B and between B and C will grow. If both presynaptic and postsynaptic neurons must fire and then rest, and only those synapses instrumental in making the postsynaptic neuron fire are strengthened, the connection from B to C will grow. Given a large number of polysynaptic pathways from A to D, the presence of stronger synapses anywhere in these pathways increases the probability that A will elicit D. Consequently, the development of a conditioned response would occur regardless of what rest principle model was used. This is also the reason that I refer often to pathways and connections rather than to neurons and synapses. Although this makes the discussion less concrete, it eliminates the necessity of specifying particular models.

The major pathways that would be expected to be involved in the development of the conditioned response, according to the rest principle, are summarized in Fig. 4.2. Other pathways, not shown for the sake of simplicity, also might have some influence. If the animal usually is fed only intermittently, as opposed to having continual access to food, S_{food} will have a strong input to R_{in} (as shown in Table 3.3). If the bell is presented only when the animal is hungry and prior to the giving of food, S_{bell} will develop connections to R_{in}, either directly, through unspecified interneurons, or via S_{food}, S_{h+food}, and S_h, in addition to the connec-

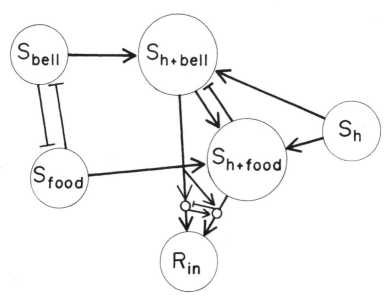

FIG. 4.2.   The major pathways involved in the development of conditioned salivation to the ringing of a bell, after the bell has been followed by the presentation of food to a hungry animal. Inhibitory connections are symbolized ⊣; facilitory connections are symbolized →.

tion via $S_{h+\text{bell}}$ shown. Lateral inhibition from S_{food} to S_{bell} and from S_{bell} to S_{food} is shown, although this has not been discussed; evidence that such inhibition exists between and within sensory systems is presented in Chapters 5 and 10.

Actually only salivation, and not the entire R_{in} response complex, is emitted. The reason for this would appear to be that the other parts of the complex require feedback from the mouth in order to coordinate the movements. You cannot chew properly unless you can feel where the food is, and neither can the dogs in the classical conditioning experiments. It would be predicted that when the bell has been rung, the animal would chew and swallow a tasteless substance placed in its mouth that it would otherwise spit out. These ideas are discussed more thoroughly at the end of this chapter.

If the bell is first paired with food, so that it elicits salivation, and then is rung continually without giving any food, $S_{h+\text{bell}}-R_{\text{in}}$ would be used continually and thus would become weaker and weaker until no salivation would be produced by the bell. Thus the conditioned response (CR) would be extinguished.

If, in the process of extinction, a pause is made in which the bell is not rung, $S_{h+\text{bell}}-R_{\text{in}}$ would be allowed to rest and thus regain some of its lost strength. When the bell is again rung, it therefore will be found to have recovered some of its ability to elicit salivation. Thus "spontaneous recovery" (Pavlov, 1927, Wagner, Siegel, Thomas, & Ellison, 1964) could be produced.

If the extinction trials are given one after another (i.e., "massed"), there will be little chance for $S_{h+\text{bell}}-R_{\text{in}}$ to rest between trials and recover its lost strength from firing. Consequently, extinction will proceed rapidly. If the trials are given at widely separated times, however, this connection will be allowed to rest for relatively long periods and may recover almost all of its strength. Thus the rest principle automatically makes massed extinction trials much more effective than spaced ones. Experimentally, this has consistently been found to be the case (e.g., Konorski, 1967, p. 37; Pavlov, 1927, pp. 52–53).

On the other hand, during the formation of conditioned responses, the rest principle states that spaced trials will be more effective because the connections will then be allowed to rest for longer periods. This advantage of spaced over massed trials in acquisition has also been found in a wide variety of learning experiments.

The rate of extinction should also be dependent on how consistently reinforcement is given during acquisition. Normally, circuits that excite themselves will reverberate after being stimulated and thus quickly weaken their connections. If, however, reinforcement is presented on every acquisition trial, self-exciting circuits within the $S_{h+\text{bell}}-R_{\text{in}}$ pathway will be prevented from self-destructing by the lateral inhibition from the pathways involved in eating. Then during extinction, when this inhibition does not follow, the self-exciting circuits will reverberate after the bell is rung, weakening their own connections and, through their output, weakening the remaining portions of the pathway. In contrast, if there are some nonreinforced trials during acquisition, most of the self-exciting circuits within $S_{h+\text{bell}}-R_{\text{in}}$ will have been eliminated before the extinction trials begin. Consequently, including nonreinforced trials during acquisition (i.e., "partial reinforcement") will tend to make the response harder to extinguish. There are, however, other factors, such as the development of self-inhibitory connections (see Chapter 5), that could either contribute to or counteract this "partial reinforcement effect," depending on the circumstances.

A computer simulation has been conducted to show how the rest principle predicts that animals should behave during classical conditioning and extinction. In this simulation, connections not used during a cycle become stronger by the amount $m^2 e^{-m}$, whereas connections that are used on this cycle become weaker by this amount: m is the number of cycles since the connection was last used. In other words, firing causes a connection to become more plastic by setting $m = 1$ and thus making it susceptible to more change on subsequent cycles. If it rests on these cycles, it becomes stronger, but the size of the increment in strength becomes smaller as m increases beyond 2.

The only effect of reinforcement (i.e., giving food) is to reduce the percentage of the connections involved in producing the CR that continue firing on each successive cycle after the presentation of the CS. This percentage also varies as a function of the strength of the connections themselves, as might be expected: The stronger the connections, the higher the percentage of connections that continue being used on each successive cycle.

Figure 4.3 compares the results from simulations of acquisition of a conditioned response with massed and with spaced trials. When the CS–UCS trials (X) were spaced by 14 time cycles, the response strength, as determined by the mean strength of the connections involved in producing the CR, grew rapidly to a high asymptotic level. When the CS–UCS trials (O) were separated by only 4 time cycles, however, learning was much poorer.

Figure 4.4 compares the results from simulations of extinction of a conditioned response with massed and with spaced trials. Massed trials now are more effective than are spaced trials.

This superiority of spaced trials in acquisition and massed trials in extinction is an automatic corollary of the rest principle: Spaced trials cause the connections to be used infrequently and thus increase the chances that they can rest and get stronger; massed trials cause them to be used more often and thus increase the chances that habituation will occur and the connections will become weaker.

This distinction between acquisition and extinction presents problems, however, for the use principle. The use principle alone allows connections only to become stronger. Extinction, therefore, cannot be attributed to a weakening of connections. The addition of the disuse principle does not change this conclusion, because the connections are being used very frequently during massed extinction trials. Consequently, extinction usually has been seen as just another form of acquisition: either learning to do something else than the CR or learning not to make the previously acquired response. It is therefore very difficult for use

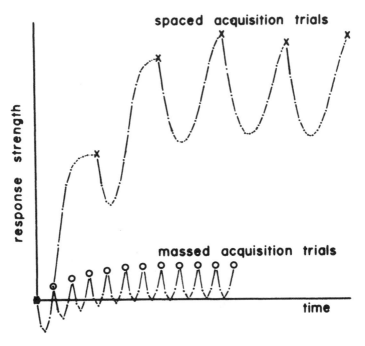

FIG. 4.3. Results from simulations of the acquisition of a conditioned response, based upon the rest principle. According to this principle, the strength of the connections involved in producing the CR, and consequently the response strength, grows as a function of the percentage of the connections that are allowed to rest after being fired during the trial. Presentation of the UCS is seen as increasing this percentage. In these simulations, 20% initially started resting after each successive time cycle. The percentage became smaller, however, after the later trials, as the connections grew stronger, thus resulting in the response strengths going to asymptotes. Massed trials resulted in the connections being used again, before they had had much time for resting and growing stronger. Consequently, the massed trials were less effective than spaced trials in acquisition.

principle theories to account for the fact that acquisition and extinction are obviously different, inasmuch as spaced trials are more effective in the former and massed trials in the latter.

Returning to Fig. 4.4: When a long interval was introduced between CS presentations after several massed extinction trials, the response strength was found to increase greatly. This spontaneous recovery occurred in the simulation for two reasons: First, rest was possible during the long interval; second, the strength of the connections had been greatly reduced by the preceding extinction trials, thus reducing reverberation, increasing the percentage of connections that could rest during the intertrial interval, and assuring that a large percentage of them would become stronger.

In the preceding pages we have been dealing with the effects of varying the intertrial interval. Now let us look at the interval between the ringing of the bell (CS) and the presentation of food (UCS). If the CS is presented before the UCS is given, the connections involving the CS (e.g., $S_{bell}-S_{h+bell}$, $S_{bell}-R_{in}$, and $S_{h+bell}-R_{in}$) should be briefly active and then should be inhibited by the activity in the pathways involving the UCS. When longer delays are used between the CS and the UCS, the CS pathways are allowed to continue firing longer and therefore will suffer some habituation before being forced to rest by inhibition from the UCS pathways and then being allowed to rest by removal of the S_h. The longer delays should thus result in poorer conditioning, as has been found (see Mackintosh, 1974, pp. 62–66).

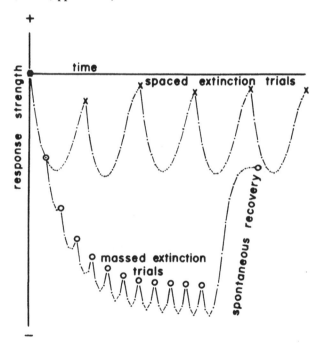

FIG. 4.4.   Results from simulations of extinction of a conditioned response, based upon the rest principle. The simulations were identical to those in Fig. 4.3, except that the absence of the UCS plus the higher initial strength of the connections produced more reverberation and therefore a lower percentage of the connections being allowed to rest. An initial value of 8% starting to rest after each time cycle was used, but this increased after later trials because of the decrease in the mean strength of the connections. Massed trials were more efficient than spaced trials in producing extinction, for the same reason that they were less efficient in producing acquisition in the simulations in Fig. 4.3. "Spontaneous recovery" was found when a long delay was introduced between trials, after several massed extinction trials had been given.

The computer simulation used to demonstrate the effect of the CS–UCS interval needed to be more complicated than those previously presented in this book. It is not possible to fit it into a programmable calculator such as the HP–97 without making such drastic simplifications that the nature of the simulation itself is changed. Consequently, I will have to describe the results obtained from a full-scale computer simulation.

A hundred registers were designated as *connections* (i.e., synapses) and given normally distributed thresholds with a mean of 100 and a standard deviation of 10. An initial stimulus (with a strength of 105 in this instance) was then given, and all connections with thresholds lower than or equal to the simulus were "used." Whenever a connection was used, a marker, m, associated with it was set to 1; connections that had thresholds above the stimulus and were not used had their markers increased by 1. At the end of each cycle, a percentage (P_m) of all connections with marker values of m were chosen randomly for having their thresholds changed. If they were used during that cycle, their thresholds were increased by 1; if they were not used, their thresholds were reduced by 1. The 1 $- P_m$ connections not chosen on that cycle had their thresholds remain unchanged. The amount of change in the mean threshold thus was a function of P_m that varied according to m: $P_m = (e^{-.4m} - e^{-.8m})$.

This formula, like that involving m in the previous simulation, reaches a maximum and then rapidly approaches zero as m increases. Thus immediately after firing a relatively large percentage of the connections are open to change, whereas after a long period of rest most of them cannot have their thresholds changed. The formula was chosen on the following grounds: Let us assume that a connection can be in one of two states only, either plastic or nonplastic. After a set of connections has been used, a process is initiated that switches them to the plastic state at a constant rate, $dx/dt = k_1x$. Those that have become plastic then return to being nonplastic at another constant rate, $dy/dt = k_2y$. The percentage in the plastic state can then be shown to be

$$\frac{k_1}{k_2 - k_1} (e^{-k_1t} - e^{-k_2t})$$

If we arbitrarily let $k_1 = .4$ and $k_2 = .8$, the percentage P_m plastic at time $t = m$ is then $e^{-.4m} - e^{-.8m}$.

After the initial stimulus, the system was seen as acting like a reverberating circuit in which the number of connections being used on cycle j, N_j, determined the stimulus, S_{j+1}, on the next cycle, according to the formula: $S_{j+1} = 60 + .60(N_j)$ during the CS–UCS interval. After the UCS was presented, inhibition from the pathways associated with it was assumed to reduce the reverberation so that $S_{j+1} = 50 + .60(N_j)$.

The results of varying the CS–UCS interval in this simulation are shown in Fig. 4.5 and 4.6. Response strength is proportional to the mean strength of the connections involved in producing the CR and thus is inversely related to their

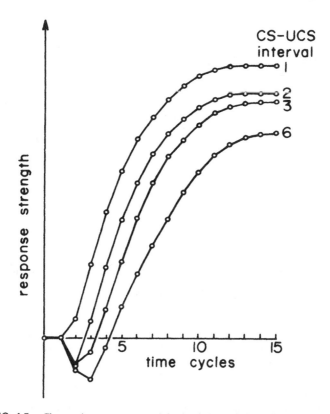

FIG. 4.5. Changes in response strength in simulations of classical conditioning, in which the UCS was introduced after 1, 2, 3, or 6 cycles of reverberation in the connections involved in producing the CR. The results are the means of 10 runs with each interval.

mean threshold. The results were rather susceptible to random variations, which show up despite the use of the means of 10 runs with each interval in these figures. Nevertheless, it still can be seen that the shorter CS–UCS intervals generally produce larger increases in response strength.

Notice that with the longer intervals, there still was some increase in response strength. In fact, an increase was found even when the UCS was never presented. This is, of course, a function of the parameters used in the simulation. Nevertheless, it is important that such increases can occur. The response strength may not be elevated high enough to elicit the CR, but still high enough so that a record is present in the subject's memory of the CS.

I dwell on this point at some length because it serves as an introduction to the general topic of memory and the effects of inhibitory interneurons, which are developed further in Chapters 9 and 10. The major point is that the strengthening

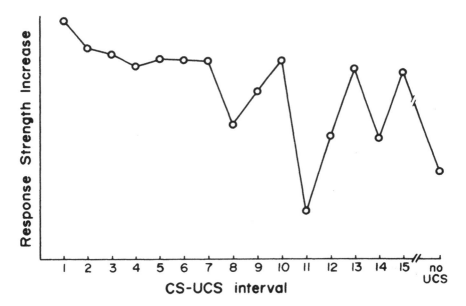

FIG. 4.6.   Mean changes in response strength in simulations of classical conditioning after 15 cycles with different CS–UCS intervals (measured in cycles). The shorter intervals produced larger (and more consistent) increases in strength. The results are the means of 10 runs with each interval.

of connections according to the rest principle allows for the production of memories of all events, regardless of whether they were reinforced or not. The ubiquitousness of memory traces becomes most apparent in the few occasions when they are not produced. A rather common situation in which this occurs is after large amounts of alcohol have been consumed, causing a "blackout." The next day, when we try to recall what happened, we find a blank interval, a period of time in which we have little or no memory of what occurred.

A similar type of amnesia occurs much more frequently, so frequently in fact that we take it for granted. We have a blackout every night when we are asleep. The blackout appears to be complete for the periods of slow-wave sleep but is more noticeable for periods of paradoxical sleep when one is dreaming. Most people have several dream periods every night, but very few dreams are ever remembered. As shown in Chapter 10, both phases of sleep probably involve inactivation of inhibitory interneurons and a special norepinephrine system that otherwise prevents spontaneous firing by the major neurons of the cerebral cortex.

A failure to store information also occurs with lack of attention. This may be partly because the sensory systems fail to transmit the information but probably also involves more central mechanisms; that is, the words, for instance, may be heard and understood but not remembered, because one was not paying attention to them. Lack of attention probably also involves reduced activity in both the inhibitory interneurons and the norepinephrine system in the cortex (see Chapter 10). Although the data are inconclusive, alcoholic blackouts may also involve these factors.

From these examples, it should be clear that the normal production of our daily memories may depend on the suppression of firing, particularly reverberatory firing, in the major neurons of the cortex. The reason for this can be seen in the preceding simulation. The degree of strengthening was an inverse function of the amount of reverberation that occurred. When the reverberation was low enough, the strengthening occurring subsequently during rest was more than sufficient to overcome the weakening occurring during the reverberation. This apparently would be an appropriate model for the cortex when the inhibitory interneurons and norepinephrine system are active. In a similar simulation but with higher initial rates of reverberation, a relationship similar to that shown in Fig. 4.6 was found but shifted lower, so no increase was found when only the CS was presented. This would be a more appropriate model for the cortex during sleep and low attention or for brain areas with fewer inhibitory interneurons and little norepinephrine input.

By varying the neuronal organization in simple ways the brain would therefore be able to obtain a variety of functions from the rest principle. For instance, one system could record events in a neutral fashion, independent of reinforcement, whereas another could have its connections strengthened only by external contingencies (e.g., finding food when the animal is hungry) and act as a sort of decision module. We discuss this theme in greater detail in Chapters 9 and 10.

Now let us return to the CS–UCS interval. Previously it was shown in the simulations that the rest principle predicts that shorter intervals produce larger increases in response strength. This relationship, however, would be expected to be true only within certain limits; the rest principle does *not* predict that the increase continues to grow as the interval becomes very short. Instead, it predicts that conditioning should be optimal at some relatively short interval and that further reductions in the interval would reduce the increase until little or no increment would be seen when the CS and UCS begin simultaneously. The reason for this is quite simple: The rest principle requires that the connections be used at least once before resting in order for the strength to be increased. After some point, as the CS–UCS interval becomes shorter and shorter, progressively fewer connections will be used before being inhibited by output from the UCS pathways. In the extreme case in which the CS and UCS begin at the same time, it is possible that the CS would be able to excite none of the connections before the inhibition came, and then no increase in strength would occur. This prediction is in agreement with the experimental data (Bitterman, 1964; Mackintosh, 1974, p. 57; Smith, Coleman, & Gormezano, 1969).

The finding that beginning the CS and UCS simultaneously does not produce significant conditioning appears to be contrary to the predictions from several previous theories. For instance, Hebb (1949) postulated that "any two cells or systems of cells that are repeatedly active *at the same time* will tend to be 'associated,' so that activity in one facilitates activity in the other [p. 70, italics mine]." Consequently, Hebb's formulation seems to suggest that the best conditioning would occur with simultaneous beginning of the CS and UCS.

It might be argued that for the production of a CR the systems that need to be active "at the same time" are those involved with the CS and UCR rather than the CS and UCS. This, however, would require that the UCS precede the CS, and such "backward conditioning" has generally been found to be ineffective (see Mackintosh, 1974, pp. 58–60).

The present theory also predicts that backward conditioning should not work. Nothing occurs after the presentation of the CS to inhibit reverberation. Any inhibition remaining from firing within the UCS pathways would prevent the initial activation of CS pathways at the same time that it would inhibit reverberation. One trivial exception to this would be if the UCS had a delayed action. For instance, the nausea produced by lithium develops some time after the injection, so the drug could be given before the CS, and conditioned aversion would still be produced.

The same simulation used to test the effect of the CS–UCS interval was also used to determine the influence of CS intensity according to the rest principle. The CS–UCS interval was kept constant at 4 cycles and the initial stimulus intensity varied between 70 and 120 (instead of being kept constant at 105, as previously). The results are shown in Fig. 4.7. Up to 105, stronger CS intensities produce greater increases in response strength, as has been found experimentally (see Mackintosh, 1974, pp. 41–45). Increasing the CS intensity above 105 caused a decrease in conditioning. This is in agreement with Pavlov's "law of strength" and with the results from some Russian studies (Razran, 1957) but not with the findings of Kamin and Brimer (1963) who saw no decrease with very intense stimuli. It might be mentioned that the CS intensity of 110 often was "painful" and those above 110 always were "painful." What is meant by "painful" is discussed more fully in Chapters 7 and 8. Briefly, unpleasantness and pain are seen as occurring whenever connections are becoming weaker: The greater the rate of decrease in strength, the greater the unpleasantness. In the present simulation, the computer was programmed to say "OUCH" whenever the mean strength was reduced on a cycle by more than a given level and to say "AH!" whenever it was increased by more than this amount. No comments were made at an intensity of 105. At 110, OUCH was said at the beginning of half of the runs and AH! later on in these runs; AH! was the only comment in the remaining runs. At intensities above 110, OUCH was always said at the beginning of the run when the CS was given and during the next few cycles while there still was high reverberation, followed by AH!s on the next cycle or two.

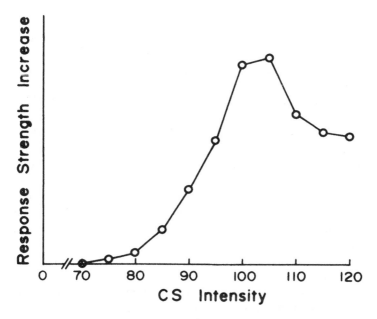

FIG. 4.7.   Results from a simulation of classical conditioning, based upon the rest principle, in which the intensity of the CS was varied. The 100 "connections" in the simulation had normally distributed thresholds with a mean of 100 arbitrary units and a standard deviation of 10. The abscissa in this figure is scaled in the same arbitrary units. The mean asymptotic levels of the response strength increases (after 28 cycles) for 10 runs are shown.

What would happen if the UCS, rather than the CS, produced OUCH comments? In most of the examples mentioned so far, we have considered an appetitive, pleasant UCS (i.e., food for a hungry animal). It is well-known that conditioning can be produced also by aversive, unpleasant UCSs, such as electric shock, air puffs, and loud noises. When we contrast instrumental and classical conditioning, there appears to be a similarity for pleasant reinforcers: In both cases the pathways that have just fired before the presentation of such stimuli become stronger. A paradox seems to occur, however, in the case of aversive reinforcers. In instrumental learning, the pathways that fire before such unpleasant stimuli are given become weaker (e.g., an animal stops doing those things that produce shock). In classical conditioning, on the other hand, the pathways that fire before an aversive UCS is presented seem to become stronger.

Upon closer examination this paradox disappears. The critical factor in classical conditioning is not the level of firing of the neurons in all regions (as it is in instrumental learning) but rather the difference between the firing rate in the region near the UCS–UCR pathway and the rate in all other regions. In the present model it is the inhibition from the strongly firing UCS–UCR pathway that causes this difference and thus causes the connections from the CS to the UCS–UCR pathway to become stronger than the connections from the CS to other responses. Before training, the responses connected to the CS are in equilibrium, and therefore no response emerges. (Or at least, CR is not the strongest of the responses and so does not appear.) The CR develops when this equilibrium is destroyed, and the connections from the CS to the CR are stronger than those to other responses. This could happen equally well by having: (1) all pathways becoming stronger, but the increment being greatest in the CS–CR connections; or (2) all pathways becoming weaker, but the decrement being smallest in CS–CR. The former would be the case with very pleasant UCSs. Pleasantness is defined in this theory as the state that occurs when the mean strength of the connections is increasing. The latter (2) would be the case for unpleasant UCSs, inasmuch as unpleasantness is defined as the state occurring when the mean strength of the connections is decreasing.

If we suppose that the ratio between the specific UCS–UCR excitation and the diffuse excitation remains constant for any one type of UCS, the absolute difference between the two would increase as a function of the UCS intensity. Because this difference determines conditioning, it would be expected that within a particular paradigm the growth of the CR would be an direct function of the UCS intensity, as has been found experimentally (see Mackintosh, 1974, pp. 70, 71). Certainly it is clear that if the UCS has an intensity of zero, the difference between the two types of excitation elicited by the UCS will also be zero, and conditioning will not occur.

Earlier it was mentioned that the CR is not identical to the UCR. In the typical example used here, the CR consists primarily of salivation and does not show the entire R_{in} seen in the UCR (for instance, chewing and swallowing do not occur). A likely reason for this is that eating is not a simple unitary response but rather a complex response chain involving the sequential interaction of stimuli and responses. The response chain is believed to be produced by a hierarchical organization, such as shown in Fig. 4.8. In this figure, the most general stimuli are shown at the top and the most specific at the bottom. Each junction in the diagram consists of a relatively general stimulus above and at least two more specific stimuli below: The latter include the general simulus but differ from one another as to a factor not specified by the more general stimulus. For instance, at one junction at the bottom of the diagram the general stimulus is

$$S_{h \, +\text{food stimuli} \atop +\text{food in mouth} \atop +\text{dry and hard}}$$

This is supposed to represent a set of neurons that have the *potential* for being fired only when a hungry animal has dry hard food in its mouth. Within this set are two subsets of neurons that require additional input before firing. One subset

(A) fires only when the animal's jaw is up, whereas the other (B) fires only when the jaw is down, in addition to meeting the other stimulus requirements. These subsets are represented in the diagram by the two specific stimuli listed below the more general stimulus. Each subset is connected to the response that eliminates its specific stimulus.

Now let us suppose that a hungry animal with dry hard food in its mouth has its jaw up. The subset (A) of neurons stimulated by these conditions fires,

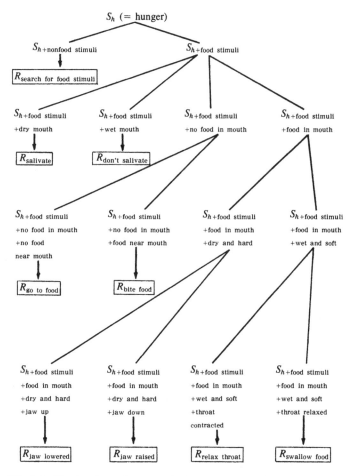

FIG. 4.8 Simple scheme for the production of the response chain involved in eating. A hungry animal searches for stimuli associated with food. When it finds some, it begins salivating and goes to the food. Once it is close enough to the food, it takes a bite, chews it, and then swallows, thus eventually reducing hunger. Notice that each response removes the specific stimulus that elicited it: Consequently this scheme would develop automatically according to to the rest principle.

causing the animal to lower its jaw. The stimuli are now no longer appropriate for subset (A), and they stop firing, with the help of inhibition from subset (B) whose required stimulus conditions are now met. So (B) fires, causing the jaw to be raised and reinstating the stimuli needed for (A). Thus the animal will continue alternately raising and lowering its jaw, until finally the food is no longer dry and hard but rather wet and soft. Now the stimuli are not correct for either subset (A) or (B) or indeed for any of the original set of neurons. So all the cells in this set will rest, with the help of inhibition from the set of neurons stimulated when a hungry animal has wet soft food in its mouth.

All the junctions in the diagram operate in a manner similar to this. By tracing through the diagram it is possible to see roughly how the response chain involved in eating would be produced. This is, of course, a simplification. Particularly on the left side of the figure the responses could have been divided and subdivided into finer and finer components.

According to this scheme, then, the reason why chewing and swallowing do not occur as part of the CR is that stimulus conditions are not correct for producing these responses: Stimuli from the presence of food in the mouth are missing. Furthermore, the detailed characteristics of this stimulus are missing. The animal cannot decide whether to chew or swallow the food unless there is information about the consistency of the food. This may be clearer to you if you have ever tried eating after having been given a local anesthetic by your dentist. Chewing is possible, but it is no longer an automatic activity and must be done with a great deal of careful conscious effort.

Salivation, on the other hand, does not require such stimuli coming from the presence of food in the mouth. There is no teleological reason for this to be so. Chewing without such input can lead to biting off one's tongue or at least to not chewing correctly. It is almost impossible to salivate incorrectly, and it is probably advantageous to salivate before the food enters the mouth. Similarly, going to the food or, for a restrained dog, orienting to the place where food usually is presented does not require stimulation from the presence of food in the mouth and therefore, like salivation, should be seen as part of the CR.

This scheme is not particularly new or unique to the present theory. What is unique, however, is that the theory shows how such an organization would develop automatically: Any population of neurons with diffuse random input from the required stimuli and diffuse random outputs to the responses would become organized in this way if they operated according to the rest principle.

In order to produce the organization seen in Fig. 4.8, each specific stimulus should become strongly connected only to the response that eliminates this stimulus. This response is therefore the one that would allow the connections to it to rest and become stronger, as dictated by the rest principle. The development is thus the same as those we have encountered several times previously.

More specifically: Imagine that the neurons fired by the combination of hunger + food in mouth + dry and hard + jaw up initially had outputs of various strengths to all the responses shown in the figure and to numerous other responses. If any of the responses other than lowering the jaw are made, the stimulation remains and the connections would become weaker by habituation. Several of the responses actually would result in an increase in the stimuli exciting these neurons, and these would be habituated very rapidly. Once the response of lowering the jaw is made, however, the neurons stop firing, and the connections from them to this response grow stronger. Subsequently, after raising the jaw has also been partially learned and the dry hard food has been made into wet soft food, the connections are further allowed to rest while swallowing is occurring and while the next bite is being sought and taken. Finally, the elimination of hunger itself will assure a very long period of rest.

The appropriate inhibitory connections between opponent stimulus–response systems would also develop automatically according to the rest principle and would further contribute to the strengthening of the correct facilitory connections. This process is discussed in Chapter 5.

5 Lateral Inhibition

I use the term *lateral inhibition* collectively for a class of neuronal organizations, including *reciprocal lateral inhibition, recurrent inhibition,* and *feed-forward lateral inhibition.* Within a system of parallel pathways, as shown in Fig. 5.1, if the output from B inhibits its neighbors A and C, and B in turn is inhibited by their output, the organization will be called *reciprocal lateral inhibition.* If, *in addition,* the output from B also inhibits the firing of B itself, the organization is called *recurrent inhibition. Feed-forward lateral inhibition* is present in a system in which the output from b inhibits A and C, whereas the outputs from a and c inhibit B.

Lateral inhibition can be extremely useful. (This is particularly true in a nervous system built with the rest principle as introduced in Chapter 4 and as seen in later chapters.) In sensory systems it can sharpen the input, increasing the contrast between adjacent or similar stimuli and elevating the signal-to-noise ratio. In motor output systems it can also focus the information, helping to reduce noise caused by output to other pathways. Furthermore, it can eliminate the tonic stimulation of one muscle when the opposing muscle is activated; thus, because of lateral inhibition, contraction of a flexor usually is accompanied by relaxation

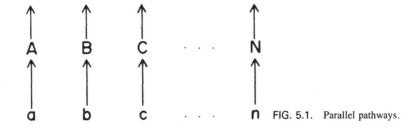

FIG. 5.1.   Parallel pathways.

of the opposing extensor, producing a greater and more efficient response. Similarly, at higher levels, it can eliminate competition between opposing responses. For instance, in an emergency situation both "fight" and "flight" responses may be partially activated. Without lateral inhibition they would interfere with each other so that neither could be carried out effectively. Lateral inhibition, however, allows the stronger response completely to dominate the weaker. It seems likely that a similar process involving lateral inhibition is important in directing attention. Computer simulations also have shown that lateral inhibition can be beneficial in memory storage and retrieval (Kohonen, Lehtiö, Rovamo, Hyvärinen, Bry, & Vainio, 1977), increasing the capacity and selectivity of a distributed network memory.

Considering the potential usefulness of lateral inhibition, it is not surprising that it occurs in many neuronal systems. It is perhaps best known in the visual sensory system but exists in other sensory systems as well. It is used in the organization of peripheral motor output and, at higher motor levels, in the cerebellum. The presence of lateral inhibition in the hippocampus is well documented (Eccles, 1967) and is known to exist in the cerebral cortex (Creutzfeldt, Kuhnt, & Benveneto, 1974; Hess, Negishi, & Creutzfeldt, 1975). Within these systems it is extremely general and widespread. Elsewhere the evidence is less conclusive, but lateral inhibition does seem to be found as a local phenomenon.

It is clear that the widespread prevalence of lateral inhibition could be the result of evolutionary selection: Animals possessing it would have a distinct advantage over those who did not. This raises the problem of how lateral inhibition develops (i.e., What is the genetic information causing lateral inhibition that is selected by evolution?). The most uneconomical process would be for every neuron to be directed to its target by the genetic code, so that the proper inhibitory interneurons would grow between the pathways and would be innervated appropriately by the neurons in the pathway. Indeed, the amount of genetic material needed to direct specifically the billions of neurons would probably be greater than the total capacity of the nucleus. A compromise solution would be to have general rules encoded about what types of neurons can innervate what other types (e.g., to have facilitory neurons innervate only inhibitory interneurons and inhibitory interneurons innervate only the facilitory neurons in the pathways). There are, however, several systems in which this particular rule is known to be violated. Any similar rule that could correctly produce the known lateral inhibitory systems would have to be very complicated and would therefore require a large amount of genetic material. Additional material would also be needed to produce the topological relationships found between different levels in the pathways, such as the way in which a map of the retina is reproduced at lower levels in the visual system, and a map of the body surface is recreated in the tactual sensory cortex.

A third alternative, by far the most parsimonious, for the production of lateral inhibition would be to have the synapses of all neurons become stronger when the conditions produced by a lateral inhibitory organization were present and to become weaker under other conditions. As is shown later, a characteristic of lateral inhibitory networks is that the firing rates of all neurons is kept at a moderately low level even when the input is high. In networks with other types of organizations, the firing rates of at least some of the neurons become very high when the input rate is elevated. Therefore, lateral inhibition would develop if synapses became stronger when they fired relatively infrequently and weaker when they fired too often in a given period of time. This is, of course, the rest principle. Furthermore, as shown at the end of this chapter, not only would neurons employing the rest principle automatically develop a lateral inhibition organization under most circumstances: The principle also favors the crossing over of nerves found between the brain and the body and the topological mapping found in the primary projection areas.

Let us now consider in more detail how rest principle neurons will develop lateral inhibition. Our starting point will be a system of parallel pathways conveying information from $a, b, c, \ldots, n$ through $A, B, C, \ldots, N$ as shown in Fig. 5.1. At the level of $A, B, C, \ldots, N$ we will let interneurons grow, without any specifications. Both facilitory and inhibitory neurons may be present and the growth can be random, so that all possible organizations may start to develop. Our only assumption will be that the input from $a, b, c, \ldots, n$ will at times be very high: As an example we will have them firing 90% of the time, using an unspecified unit of time. The various organizations will be examined, beginning with those that would habituate most rapidly according to the rest principle and ending with those favored by this principle.

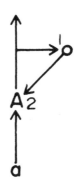

FIG. 5.2.   Self-facilitation.

As shown in Fig. 5.2, after the first time that a gives an input to A, the connections 1 and 2 will have their presynaptic and postsynaptic parts active half of the time, as the wave of excitations reverberates around the small two-neuron loop. As soon as another input from a reaches A during a cycle when it would not otherwise be firing, the connections 1 and 2 would be active on every cycle. Such continual firing would rapidly weaken these connections.

Figure 5.3 demonstrates that if any input comes to either B or C, a reverberating circuit is begun. For instance, if b fires B, then B will fire x, x will fire C, C

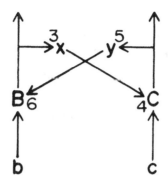

FIG. 5.3.   Reciprocal facilitation.

will fire y, y will fire B, and so on. In a four-neuron loop such as this, all units initially would be firing 25% of the time. As new inputs come to B and C out of phase with the initial firing of the circuit, a second, third, and fourth wave of excitation would be started in the loop, eventually making all units fire on every cycle. This will take a little longer than it did in the two-neuron loop of self-facilitation, but if the input rates from both b and c are 90%, the probability is .65 that all units will be firing already on the second cycle. Connections 3, 4, 5, and 6 would then habituate rapidly. Even with very low rates of input, the neurons will eventually be firing all the time and the connections will grow weaker.

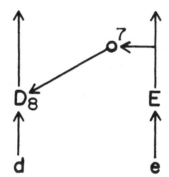

FIG. 5.4.   One-way facilitation.

The organization shown in Fig. 5.4 avoids the problem of reverberating circuits found in the first two arrangements. Consequently, unlike them it will not become nonfunctional if the input is restricted to low rates. However, if the input increases, say to 90% of the time, to both D and E from d and e, connection 7 will have both presynaptic and postsynaptic parts firing 90% of the time, whereas connection 8 will have its presynaptic neuron firing 90% and its postsynaptic neuron 99% of the time. If the critical percentage for maintaining synaptic strength (i.e., $1 - P_c$) is much lower than 90%, both connections would rapidly become weaker.

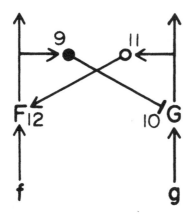

FIG. 5.5.   One-way facilitation and one-way inhibition.

An exact determination of the firing rates of F and G as shown in Fig. 5.5, is rather complicated because the rate for each is dependent on the rate for the other. A close approximation can be obtained with

$$F = p + (1-p)\left\{p\left[\ \frac{p}{p + p + (1-p)(.5p)}\ \right]\right\}$$

$$G = p\left(\frac{p}{p + p + (1-p)\left\{p\left[\ \frac{p}{p + p + (1-p)(.5p)}\ \right]\right\}}\right)$$

where p is the input rate from both e and f. If $p = 90\%$, F would fire 94.39% and G, 43.93% of the time. If both presynaptic and postsynaptic factors contribute to the changes in synaptic strength, of the four connections involving interneurons, connection 9 would be the first to weaken because both parts would be firing 94.39% of the time. Once it becomes nonfunctional, the organization is the same as that with D and E (i.e., one-way facilitation), and then connections 11 and 12 would also be rapidly weakened.

All-or-none output, such as used in the simulations reported in Table 5.1, reduces the firing of G. A separate simulation with graded outputs showed that

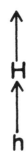

FIG. 5.6.   No connections.

when the input rate was 90%, over 1000 cycles F fired 94.7% and G, 42.2% of the time.

Inasmuch as we are considering the connections with interneurons in this section, there is little to say about such an isolated pathway as h - H, shown in Fig. 5.6. However, the firing rate within the pathway will be high when h produces a rapid input, and therefore the connections within the pathway itself will habituate. This is covered when we discuss the strength of the connections within the pathways, later in this chapter.

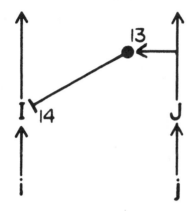

FIG. 5.7.   One-way inhibition.

If i and j are firing 90% of the time, as in Fig. 5.7, both presynaptic and postsynaptic units for connection 13 and the presynaptic part of 14 also will fire 90% of the time. The postsynaptic part of 14 will fire whenever i has an output and j did not (2 cycles earlier) and when both i and j have had outputs but output at i is greater: 9% + .5(81%) = 49.5% of the time.

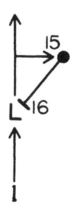

FIG. 5.8.   Self-inhibition.

Simulations have shown that the firing rate in Fig. 5.8 is dependent on whether the neurons have a graded output or an all-or-none output. In the former case, the neurons fired 65.5% of the time in a run of 1000 cycles when the input rate was 90%. In the latter, the firing rate was 46.4% when temporal summation was included and 47.6% when no temporal summation occurred. Increasing the strength of the inhibition in the graded-output simulation lowered the firing rate toward that found with all-or-none output.

Although these rates are not as high as were seen in the previous organizations, it seems likely that they are still high enough that connections 15 and 16 probably would not increase very much in strength.

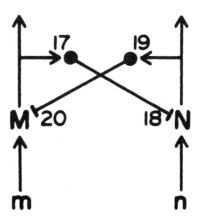

FIG. 5.9.   Reciprocal lateral inhibition.

In Fig. 5.9, we see an organization that would be viable for high input rates, according to the rest principle. The firing rate here is dependent on the extent to which the parameters are conducive to one pathway dominating for relatively long periods of time. When the parameters favor domination, the firing rate approaches:

$$\frac{1 - (1-p)^n}{n}$$

where p is the input rate and n is the number of pathways inhibited by the output of each pathway. The mean firing rate for larger networks will be increased somewhat if the parameters are such that dominance is often shared by more than one pathway or if dominance is maintained for only a few cycles and there are many periods when several pathways are vying for dominance.

The mean firing rate is relatively insensitive to changes in p. Instead, it is determined to a large extent by the size of the network, n. Therefore, connections involving the interneurons would become stronger under a wide range of input situations and the network would expand. Because the rest principle requires that a connection be activated before resting in order to become stronger, the expansion would not continue indefinitely; rather, the number of pathways included should expand to a relatively fixed limit (as has been found, for instance, in the cerebellum [Eccles, 1967]).

Over long periods of time, the mean firing rate for all neurons would be similar, and therefore all the connections involving the inhibitory interneurons would have both their presynaptic and postsynaptic units firing at the same low level. There would be no "weak links" that continually were being fired too much and that would become permanently weakened, as in the case with one-way inhibition and with one-way facilitation and one-way inhibition. There still is some danger of temporary habituation here. Once one pathway has gained complete control of the network, it will continue to dominate until (1) it fails to receive input, (2) an exceptionally strong input is received by some other pathway, or (3) the connections stimulated by it habituate. Consequently, if relatively homogeneous continuous input is fed into the system, habituation of the initially dominant pathway will occur. Once it has lost control of the system, the connections it has stimulated will recover during the long period when it is being dominated by other pathways. In the interim, however, this pathway would be relatively nonfunctional.

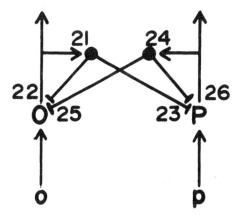

FIG. 5.10.   Recurrent inhibition.

The organization in Fig. 5.10 combines reciprocal lateral inhibition and self-inhibition: The output of each pathway inhibits all other pathways and also inhibits its own subsequent firing. With only two pathways, the firing rates are somewhat lower than with reciprocal lateral inhibition, averaging about one-third of the input rate. With a larger number of pathways, simulations have shown that if the parameters are not conducive to long-term domination, the firing rates are similar to those produced by reciprocal lateral inhibition. With recurrent inhibition none of the pathways can dominate the others for very long, and therefore none of them will habituate and become temporarily nonfunctional.

It would therefore appear that recurrent inhibition has an advantage over reciprocal lateral inhibition and that consequently the latter should be unlikely to develop. Indeed, the self-inhibitory connection that differentiates the two should be a very probable one to develop. Each pathway neuron (e.g., *P* in Fig. 5.10) is closer to the inhibitory interneuron it excites than are all other pathway neurons (e.g., *0*). Moreover, it is certain to have fired just before being inhibited and therefore would be very plastic, so the inhibitory connection could grow.

It was discovered, however, in the simulations presented in the next section, that there are situations in which reciprocal lateral inhibition produces lower, and apparently closer to optimal, firing rates than recurrent inhibition and hence would be favored by the rest principle. In most of the simulations, the threshold for firing the inhibitory neurons was .5 (arbitrary units). Lowering the threshold to .3 did not make the two types of lateral inhibition differ from each other, but when the threshold was raised to .8, reciprocal lateral inhibition produced a lower mean firing rate, 30.21%, than did recurrent inhibition, 41.11% (10 pathways, 90% inputs, 1000 cycles). The reason for this was clear when runs of only 100 cycles were used: With reciprocal lateral inhibition one pathway would dominate the others for very long periods of time, lowering the firing rate toward the $[1 - (1 - p)^n]/n$ mentioned earlier. This was not clear in the means of the 1000-cycle run, because in that run several different pathways temporarily became dominant. The difference between the two types of lateral inhibition became even more pronounced when more pathways were involved and one pathway was given input more often than the others. Using 20 pathways, with reciprocal lateral inhibition the mean firing rate was 14.55%, whereas with recurrent inhibition it was 36.10%.

Therefore, in systems in which the threshold for exciting the inhibitory interneurons is raised and in which a particular signal may persist over a relatively long period of time, reciprocal lateral inhibition will be favored by the rest principle. As discussed further in Chapter 10, it is suggested that the method by which varying degrees of attention and arousal are produced involves modulating the threshold (or strength) of the inhibitory interneurons. Consequently, in systems involving attention, there probably would be long periods of time during low arousal or sleep when the threshold would be high enough to favor reciprocal lateral inhibition over recurrent inhibition. This should have a beneficial effect for a system such as the cerebral cortex in which flexibility of pathways is desirable. A system using reciprocal lateral inhibition would remain more amenable to change than would one using recurrent inhibition, because neither habituation nor rapid growth of connections is possible with recurrent inhibition. It has been suggested that reciprocal lateral inhibition does predominate in the cerebral cortex (Walley & Weiden, 1973) but the evidence is hardly conclusive.

In summary, of the various interneurons that might have grown between the pathways, only those organizations involving lateral inhibition would develop strong connections according to the rest principle if the input rate was high at times. This would happen automatically because it is characteristic of lateral inhibition networks to maintain moderately low mean firing rates in all the neurons involved, relatively independent of the input rate. Therefore, the development of lateral inhibition would be assured by genetically encoding only one simple thing (the rest principle) in all neurons.

More complex networks, involving a combination of lateral inhibition and any of the other organizations, could also develop, but the lateral inhibition would remain dominant, with stronger connections than found in the other organizations superimposed upon it.

Organizations other than lateral inhibition could also develop in a system of pathways in which the input rates always remained low. This could be assured if the input came from another system in which there was lateral inhibition, pro vided there was little convergence. The output of each individual pathway in a system with lateral inhibition is maintained at a low rate. However, if several of these pathways converge, high levels of input might again be produced and would cause the development of lateral inhibition at this level also. For instance, according to the present theory, in the visual system lateral inhibition develops at the retinal level because of the high level of input from the receptors. The output from these pathways converges, producing progressively more complex feature analyzers. The continued presence of a particular set of features would cause a high rate of firing within the feature analyzers, thus necessitating and causing the development of lateral inhibition at these higher levels. If, on the other hand, the output from the lower levels of the visual system also went to a large network in which little convergence occurred, the firing rate for any individual neuron would be low, and lateral inhibition would not develop. This might be the case, for instance, in the reticular formation.

Now let us leave the connections involving the interneurons and look at the connections within the pathways, again supposing that the input rate sometimes reaches high levels. It will be assumed for the sake of demonstration that the various organizations of interneurons have all somehow remained viable. Table 5.1 shows the mean firing rates of the pathway neurons that occurred in simulations of the different organizations as they would exist before habituation took place. The simulations assumed that temporal summation took place: Each neuron fired only if

$$\sum_t \frac{A_0}{2} + \frac{A_1}{4} + \frac{A_2}{8} + \frac{A_3}{16} + \cdots > .5$$

where A_0 is the present input into the neuron, A_1 is the input on the previous cycle, A_2 the input 2 cycles before, and so on. If a neuron fires, its output is 1; if it does not fire, its output is 0.

If only the percentage of time firing determined whether synaptic strength would increase or decrease, and the critical percentage for maintaining synaptic strength is, say, 30%, the connections in the pathways firing more rapidly than this will weaken until their firing rate is reduced to 30%. For instance, in the pathway with no lateral connections (h - H), the connections would habituate during the 90% input so that 12 consecutive inputs from h are required to fire H, because this would happen about 30% of the time. The connections in pathways with one-way facilitation would weaken to the point where no amount of firing from a single input source would suffice; only repetitive simultaneous activation

TABLE 5.1.
Mean Firing Rates of Pathway Neurons, as Percentage of Time, in
Simulations of Various Network Organizations, When They Received
Input 90% of the Time, During 1000 Cycles

Organization	Individual Pathways					Mean
A. Two parallel pathways						
Self-facilitation	99.9		99.9			99.90
Reciprocal facilitation	99.9		99.8			99.85
One-way facilitation	99.9		89.4			94.64
No lateral connections	90.4		90.7			90.55
One-way facilitation and one-way inhibition	3.0		92.2			47.60
One-way inhibition	4.0		90.9			47.45
Self-inhibition	44.9		45.2			45.05
Reciprocal lateral inhibition	47.1		45.7			46.40
Recurrent inhibition	31.4		30.1			30.75
B. Ten parallel pathways						
Self-inhibition	45.1 46.9 47.9 43.1 42.0					45.40
	45.2 46.3 45.7 45.8 46.0					
Reciprocal lateral inhibition	15.8 16.3 15.9 16.6 16.6					16.65
	16.9 15.3 17.0 16.8 19.3					
Recurrent inhibition	16.2 16.6 17.4 17.5 17.4					16.72
	16.7 17.1 16.2 15.9 16.2					
C. Twenty parallel pathways						
Reciprocal lateral inhibition						13.10
Recurrent inhibition						13.81
D. One hundred parallel pathways						
Reciprocal lateral inhibition						10.88
Recurrent inhibition						11.36

of both input sources would cause an output. The pathways with lateral inhibition would retain their low thresholds.

So far we have considered only the mean firing rate. It is likely that recurrent inhibition would also be favored by the rest principle because of the temporal pattern of firing that this organization produces. In the simulation it has been assumed that plasticity varies as a function of m, the number of cycles after firing, becoming greatest when m is small and returning toward zero as m becomes large. Firing again during this period of high plasticity causes a larger decrease in synaptic strength than firing later when the plasticity is reduced. Therefore, even if the mean firing rate is the same, pathways that fire repeatedly and then are silent for long periods would tend to become weaker than those in which firing is selectively spaced so that firing seldom if ever occurs on two consecutive cycles.

A pathway that retained reciprocal or self-facilitation, but with weakened connections so that it fired perhaps only 30% of the time, would probably fire in huge bursts (when the reverberating loops finally are activated) separated by very long periods of silence. Even a pathway with no lateral connections that has habituated so it fires infrequently would likely to fire in bursts. For instance, if it has habituated so that 12 consecutive inputs are required to fire it, the probability is .9 that it will fire on a cycle following one in which it had fired. With recurrent inhibition, however, the probability of firing on the cycle after it has just fired is lower than at any other time, because of the self-inhibitory connection. Consequently, the critical firing rate for maintaining synaptic strength would be higher in pathways with recurrent inhibition than in pathways with other organizations.

The discussion so far has shown how pathways with lateral inhibition would remain strong or become stronger and would have low thresholds, whereas other pathways would become weaker and develop very high thresholds, if there were a high rate of input. It is also possible, according to many rest principle models, for the pathways without lateral inhibition to be made completely nonfunctional when there is competition between them and pathways with lateral inhibition for innervating the same neuron. This would be dependent on this neuron's having a limited capacity for being innervated (e.g., a limited number, N, of receptor sites). Without competition from pathways having lateral inhibition, the loss of synaptic strength occurring during rapid firing would be countered by an increase in strength while the pathway is too weak to fire. Therefore it would be periodically functional. With competition, however, and with a limited number of sites, growth of the connections from the pathway with lateral inhibition would steal away sites from the habituated pathways, eventually rendering them nonfunctional. For instance, suppose first that a neuron has all N of its sites innervated by a pathway with reciprocal facilitation. During the huge burst of firing, n of these are lost, but during the subsequent rest, all of these would be regained. On the other hand, suppose that it is innervated also by a pathway with lateral inhibition. Now, each time the reciprocal-facilitation pathway loses n sites, it regains only $.5n$, and the lateral-inhibition pathway receives the other $.5n$. After N/n bursts by the pathway with reciprocal facilitation, it would have lost all its sites and never again would be able to activate the neuron. Whether this happens depends on which model of the rest principle is used. Models including presynaptic factors are likely to lead to pathways without lateral inhibition becoming completely nonfunctional when they are in competition with lateral-inhibition pathways and there is a high rate of input; models without long-term presynaptic factors would allow them to remain periodically functional.

In addition to assuring that lateral inhibition develops and that pathways with it become dominant, the rest principle, with its negative-feedback nature, also guarantees that the pathways within the lateral inhibitory system remain relatively balanced. In the simplest case, if one pathway happens to develop stronger connections than the others, its mean firing rate will be increased until the connections have weakened to the level of its neighbors. Similarly, if the input to one pathway is higher than that to its neighbors for a prolonged period of time, it will become weaker than the neighbors. If equal input is subsequently given to all pathways, the neighbors initially will dominate the pathway that originally had the stronger input. The result would be a negative aftereffect of the previous positive stimulus. For instance, in the visual system, prolonged staring at a white pattern on a black background would produce a negative afterimage (i.e., the appearance of a black pattern) when a homogenous field is viewed, as of course does happen.

The situation with reduced strength or reduced input is at first glance more complicated. It might seem that if all pathways have their strengths adjusted so that optimal growth occurs, any with less input or any that happen to develop weaker connections would become progressively weaker than the others, inasmuch as their firing rate would now be less than optimal. This would not happen, however, because the mean strength cannot be kept at the point of optimal growth. Instead, the firing rate stays at the level at which the strengths are just maintained. The reason for this is simple. If the mean strength increases, the firing rate is increased above the maintenance rate, thus reducing the strength; conversely, if the strength happens to be decreased, the firing is reduced below the maintenance rate, causing more rest and thus increasing the strength (see Fig. 5.11). This is for pathways receiving input most of the time. These conclusions would not be true for higher systems in which the individual pathways are infrequently excited. Therefore, there is no contradiction to the arguments (p. 38) concerning the continual laying down of memories, in which the firing rate was assumed to be lower, and therefore better, than the maintenance rate.

Because the mean firing rate is kept at the maintenance level, any pathway weaker than its neighbors would be resting more and would therefore become stronger until it was again equal. Any pathway receiving lower inputs than its neighbors for prolonged periods of time would develop stronger connections than its neighbors. Subsequently, when equal inputs are given to all pathways, the pathway receiving lower inputs will dominate its neighbors until its strength is again reduced to the average. Therefore, there will be negative afterimages also for negative stimuli in which the input rate from the stimulus is reduced. For instance, looking at a black object on a white background will produce an afterimage of a white object.

Furthermore, if some receptors always received lower inputs than their neighbors, as is the case, for instance, for rods and cones lying in the shadow of the retinal blood vessels, they would develop stronger connections than their neighbors, and the pathways from them would have a mean output rate equal to that from the pathways receiving normal input. Consequently, under usual conditions we would be unaware of the reduced input to these receptors. For the same reason, stabilized images on the retina would quickly become undetectable.

These same conclusions would apply to systems as a whole, as well as to parts of a system. For instance, with vision, increasing the mean input would eventually produce a weakening of connections and a return to the maintenance rate of

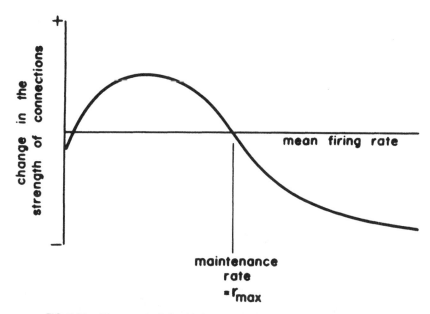

FIG. 5.11. The general relationship between the firing rate and the strengthening and weakening of connections, according to the rest principle. In frequently used pathways, a negative-feedback arrangement automatically keeps the mean firing rate near the maintenance level: Increased strength produces increased firing, which reduces strength back to the maintenance level, whereas decreased strength produces decreased firing, which increases strength back to the maintenance level.

firing, whereas decreasing the illumination would cause an eventual compensatory increase in strength. Therefore, adaptation would occur in the neural network as well as in the receptor itself. Information about changes in the general level of stimulation would reach higher levels during the transition periods while adaptation was occurring. After adaptation was completed, however, if the stimulation level were within the range where adaptation could be completed, knowledge of the general level of input would not be directly available from the current firing of the pathways with lateral inhibition and probably would have to be carried by auxiliary pathways.

It might be mentioned that practically none of these consequences of neural systems having the rest principle would occur if neurons employed the use principle. With the use principle, self-facilitation and reciprocal facilitation, with their high rates of firing, would be favored. These facilitory connections would become stronger and stronger, causing perpetual firing of the pathways involved. Because these rapidly would have reached maximum strength and would have continual input from the two- or four-neuron reverberating circuits, their output would be independent of input conditions and they would be useless as information carriers (Fig. 5.12). Any inhibitory connections would have to be pro-

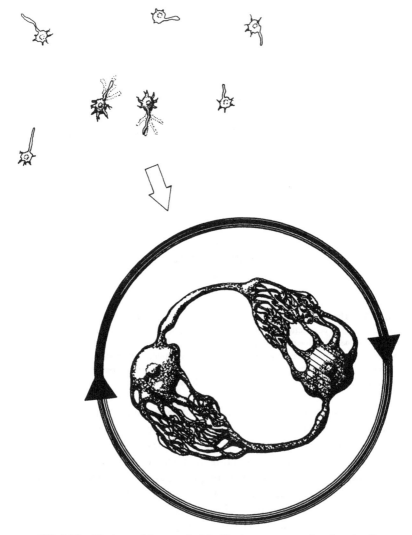

FIG. 5.12. The bane of the use principle: The two-neuron reverberating circuit.

grammed genetically and the strength of their connections assured by some process other than the use principle, because any system containing them would fire less than a system without them and thus would be overwhelmed by the purely facilitory systems. The balance between pathways also would have to be assured by some separate mechanism; otherwise, whatever pathway was strongest would fire most often and become still stronger. Permanent positive afterimages would be produced by persistent stimuli. Stabilized images on the retina would not fade but become stronger and stronger and would be seen even after they were removed.

The development of lateral inhibition, at least in the lateral geniculate of cats, does not occur until after birth and the opening of the eyes (Norman, Pettigrew, & Daniels, 1977). Furthermore, the development appears to be dependent on consistent low latencies for the arrival of input from the retina, thus causing the input to the lateral geniculate at any instant to reflect the preceding retinal firing pattern. Therefore, lateral inhibition seems to be dependent on environmentally produced input rather than on genetic preprogramming and hence would probably be controlled by factors altering the strength of connections as a function of the firing pattern. Because in the present theory these factors are postulated to operate according to the rest principle, the development of lateral inhibition is also seen as being directed by the principle. (The requirement that the input from the environment be coherent is discussed later, in the section on topological mapping.) Norman et al. (1977) also found that it was much harder to fire lateral geniculate neurons before lateral inhibition developed, agreeing with the conclusion arrived at here that low thresholds and high firing rates are necessary for the development of lateral inhibition, which in turn is necessary for the maintenance of the low thresholds.

There are two other general trends in neuronal development that also could be produced by the rest principle but that empirical evidence suggests are, at least partially, under the control of other processes. The first of these is the crossing-over of nerves between the body and the brain. This is a very general tendency. Nearly all sensory input originating on one side of the body initially projects to the other side of the brain; similarly, nearly all motor output goes from one side of the brain to the contralateral side of the body. Furthermore, input from lower parts of the body goes to upper parts of the brain, so that the connections in general for two dimensions resemble those shown in Fig. 5.13. The same pattern also can be seen somewhat in three dimensions (e.g., with the input from the eyes going to the back of the brain). The general rule appears to be that each nerve projects to a target that is farthest away from it; it may take a roundabout route, but the nerve eventually reaches the other end of the axis going through the nerve's point of origin.

The second tendency is the topological mapping in the cortex of receptor organs and the body itself. For instance, in the cortical projection of the visual system a map of the retina is produced in which adjacent retinal fields fire adjacent cortical areas. Similarly, tactual input projects so that a map of the surface of the body is created in the cortex.

Two ways in which the crossing-over could have been produced are shown in Fig. 5.14. In both it is assumed that neurons are already firing at the stage in development when the crossing over occurs, and that the firing is produced by factors that can be represented as gradients spreading periodically over the embryo. These gradients are shown in the figure by the parallel lines; the probability of firing is represented by the density of the lines.

The upper half of the figure shows how the rest principle could have produced the crossing over. The neuron has randomly grown outputs to all parts of the

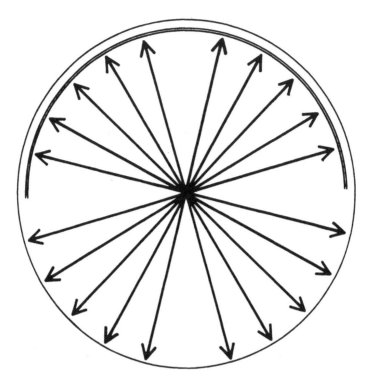

FIG. 5.13. Schematic illustrating the general crossing-over of nerves between the body (lower part of the circle) and the brain (double-lined half circle at the top). The relationship holds for both sensory input and motor output, hence the double-headed arrows.

embryo. Subsequently, those that end on targets that are likely to be fired by the gradient at the same time that they are fired by the activation of the neuron itself have their connections weakened, because they are likely to have their targets continue firing after the connection has excited the target. The target farthest away from the cell body of the neuron (O) is least likely to be fired by the gradient when the neuron is activated. Therefore, axons crossing over to the furthest point will maintain or develop strong connections with their targets, whereas others are likely to have their connections habituated.

In the lower part of the figure, a process is illustrated that is not really a part of the rest principle but could be complementary to it. Here the axon from the neuron selectively grows toward those regions in which the firing is most different from its own. A gradient coming periodically from different directions, as illustrated, would make the axon cross over and grow to the point farthest from the site of activation of the neuron itself. A set of three gradients coming from three fixed directions defining the coordinates of the embryo would have a similar effect.

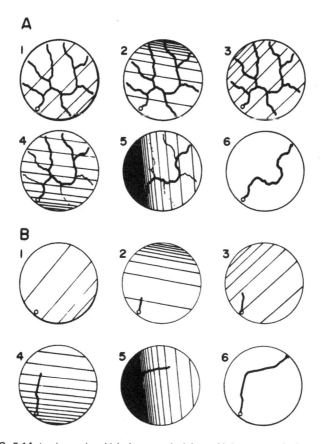

FIG. 5.14.*A* A way in which the rest principle could (but apparently does not) produce the crossing over of nerves illustrated in Fig. 5.12. The parallel lines represent gradients causing the neurons to fire. Connections are weakened whenever the gradient is exciting the cell body of the neuron itself (○) and the target neurons. Little change occurs in frames 1, 2, and 3, because the neuron is not firing rapidly. In frames 4 and 5, however, the gradients are oriented so that the neuron fires, and targets also fired by these gradients have their connections from the neuron weakened. The target farthest away from the source of activation of the neuron (which is considered here to be near the cell body) is most likely to retain strong connections. (For the sake of illustration, axon branches to weakened connections are shown to disappear, although this would not be a necessary consequence of the rest principle.

B. A process related to the rest principle, which also could (but apparently does not) cause the crossing-over, without the trial and error found in *A*. Axonal growth is postulated to go toward neurons that are stimulated by the gradient most different from the neuron itself. In frame 1, the influences from the gradient cancel each other out, but in frame 2, because there are few or no neurons behind the cell, growth proceeds toward the gradient. The amount of growth is determined by the difference in firing rate between the neurons at the tip of the axon and the neuron itself. Although both this process and the rest principle could account for the crossing-over, they are not in line with evidence suggesting that neurons maintain some information about their previous location and/or target after being transplanted.

Neither of these processes fits the empirical evidence coming from transplantation and regeneration studies (Barondes, 1975; Edds, 1967). For instance, when a piece of tissue containing Mauthner cells is tranplanted so that anterior and posterior are reversed, the cells, which normally grow posteriorly, begin growing in an anterior direction. Eventually they cross over and proceed posteriorally. The initial anterior growth suggests that the cells and the tissue retained information about their previous location, a fact that cannot be accounted for by these processes. On the other hand, the fact that the cells eventually grew posteriorally through the tissue shows that they can disregard this information. Perhaps a satisfactory explanation could be developed from the model recently proposed by French and Bryant (Bryant, Bryant, & French, 1977; French, Bryant, & Bryant, 1976; Glass, 1977) for regeneration in which maximal growth is produced when a cell encounters another whose polar coordinates were most different from its own at the time when these coordinates became a fixed label for the cells. At present, however, I know of no hypothesis that can account for all the data related to crossing-over.

The important point for the present theory is that whatever process does produce crossing-over, the end result is consistent with the rest principle. Consequently, connections established by the other processes would be maintained and strengthened if neurons operated according to this principle. The possibility also cannot be eliminated that either the rest principle or the related process shown in Fig. 5.14B may help in the establishment of these connections.

The situation is roughly similar for topological mapping. If we assume, for now, that a system of lateral inhibition already existed between the target neurons in the projection area, the rest principle could make pathways excited by adjacent skin areas or retinal areas (a, b, c, ...) develop strong connections with adjacent target neurons (A, B, C, ...). The primary reason for this is that with spatial stimuli, it is very unlikely that a stimulus will appear in one spot, then disappear, and reappear in some distant spot. Far more often a stimulus moves in a continuous fashion, thus stimulating adjacent receptors consecutively: The next receptor to fire after b is most likely to be a or c, not n. If c already has a connection to C and C inhibits B (lateral inhibition), when a connection from b to B fires B, it is likely that B will subsequently be inhibited when the stimulus moves on from b to c. A connection from b to B is very likely to be strengthened according to the rest principle. A connection from b to N will not be strengthened because N is not subjected to lateral inhibition from C.

Receptor b could as easily have developed strong connections with D, if c–C is the only existing connection. Thus this argument does not determine whether the mapping will be a–A, b–B, c–C, d–D, e–E or a–E, b–D, c–C, d–B, e–A, only that adjacent receptor fields become connected to adjacent targets. The orientation of the map must be determined by other processes. The evidence from regeneration and transplantation studies also suggests that other processes are responsible for the orientation of the map and for getting the projections into the general area of their eventual destination. Within this area, however, the point-to-point variations in the gradients apparently used by these processes must be very small, and the innervation produced would be relatively inaccurate. Nevertheless, it would provide the projection area with an input sufficient for the development of lateral inhibition. As shown in the simulations, the requirement for the development of lateral inhibition was only that the pathway neurons had a high rate of input; the input did not need to be coherent. The growth of the inhibitory connections with this relatively incoherent input would be determined primarily by distance: The interneuron excited by any particular pathway would inhibit most the pathways lying closest to it.

The development of these fields of lateral inhibition in the projection area provides the prerequisite for corrections to be made on the connections between inputs from the retinal and the target neurons, when myelinization of the input axons reduces the latencies to consistently low values, thus producing coherent input. The correction would, as described before, then lead to the topological mapping organization. As the correct connection of a to A, b to B, ..., n to N proceeded, a refinement of the lateral inhibition network is likely to occur. With proper lateral inhibitory connections (e.g., between B and C) the firing of the inhibitory neuron from B to C is likely to be quickly suppressed as the stimulus moves on from b to c, and C inhibits B. If, however, lateral inhibition had developed "incorrectly" between B and N, the inhibitory neuron from B to N might continue firing when the stimulus went from b to the adjacent receptor c. Thus the topological development of the projection connections and the lateral inhibitory connections would proceed jointly, each tending to refine the other.

As a final note to this chapter, I would like to state that the real relationship between the other processes determining embryonic neuronal development and the rest principle is intriguing but so far has been elusive. The fact that both determine the connections between neurons and that the rest principle could have produced end results that are determined by these other processes suggests that there may be a fundamental similarity between them. It would be very satisfying if one could generate the rest principle from, for instance, French and Bryant's (1976) model or, conversely, generate a totally accurate explanation of neuronal development from a modification of the rest principle. Such attempts to date have not been successful but seem very much worth pursuing. If successful, they might lead to an even more general and inclusive principle, one that could clarify the issue as to which of the rest principle models is correct.

Consistent with the ideas presented here, Changeux and Danchin (1976) have cited evidence that genetically determined factors direct the growth of axons only to the general target area; they have proposed that a trial-and-error process is important for the "selective stabilization" of the fine details of the final pattern of innervation. The latter process seems to occur primarily after birth, when large numbers of functional synapses are known to be lost. This proposition is discussed further in Chapter 6.

6 Physiological Evidence Backing the Rest Principle

As mentioned previously, the *rest principle* is not a specific physiological process. Instead, it is a general rule that neurons are postulated to obey. There are numerous processes that could cause neurons to act in accordance with the principle. In this chapter we consider the empirical data showing that such processes do exist. We first look at variations in the receptivity of the postsynaptic cell, which others (e.g., Huttunen, 1973) have postulated as being the major factor responsible for the strengthening of synapses and thus for learning.

Results in compliance with the rest principle would be produced if the responsiveness of the postsynaptic neuron decreased when the receptors were used continually and the response made repeatedly but increased when the receptors were not used and no further response was elicited after a response was once produced. (The term *response* here means the event occurring in the postsynaptic cell when enough receptors are stimulated by their agonists.) Recently there has been an avalanche of reports showing that this is precisely how most receptors do function. Variation is still present. In some systems, change is produced by varying the number of receptors; in other systems, the affinity of the receptors to transmitter is altered; and in still others it appears that the ability of receptors to produce their response is changed.

Receptors are found on all cells, not just on neurons, and the nonneuronal receptors have been studied more thoroughly. Excellent evidence is also available for the changes in nonneuronal receptors to substances that are believed to be transmitters for neurons. Fewer results have been obtained concerning the receptors on neurons, but these are in agreement with the other work.

In 1957, Beale showed that the number of surface antigens (i.e., receptors) on *Paramecia* was decreased when large numbers of antibodies were present. It was

66

believed that this happened because the antibodies caused the organism to shed the antigens. The disappearance of antigens after antibodies are introduced has since been found with thymus–leukemia antigens, H-2 antigens, and immunoglobulin molecules (Boyse, Old, & Luell, 1963) and is called *antigenic modulation*. The loss of antigens is caused by pinocytosis of the antibody–antigen complex; that is, the surface membrane invaginates, surrounding the complex, and then pinches off to form a vesicle inside the cell. The number of antigens lost is a function of the antibody concentration. After 6–24 hours in which no antibodies are present, the number of antigens returns to normal, provided that protein synthesis is not inhibited. Thus, in accordance with the requirements of the rest principle, excessive filling of these receptors causes a reduction in their number, whereas a period of rest without any filling causes an increase.

A roughly similar picture has emerged for hormone receptors. The story started with the recognition (Berson & Yalow, 1964) that many diabetics who acquired the condition in maturity showed an insensitivity to insulin. Instead of being insulin-deficient, these patients often were found to have elevated insulin levels. Initially it was thought they might have had an insulin inhibitor, but none has been found (Roth, Neville, Kahn, & Gorden, 1977). Instead, these diabetics had a reduced number of insulin receptors (Bar, Gorden, Roth, Kahn, & De-Meyts, 1976; Harrison, Martin, & Melick, 1976; Olefsky, 1976). Furthermore, with the proper diet program for reducing the insulin level, the number of receptors could be increased.

Parallel findings have been made in genetically obese mice. These animals also have an elevated level of insulin and are insulin-resistant. As with the human diabetic, these symptoms are associated with a striking reduction in the number of insulin receptors. On hepatocytes, adipocytes, thymocytes, and muscles, 50 to 70% reductions are found (Kahn, 1976), although there is some disagreement regarding the adipocytes (Maugh, 1976). The remaining receptors have been reported to have a normal affinity for insulin (Soll, Kahn, & Neville, 1975), although others, as discussed later, have reported that high levels of insulin reduce the affinity of the receptors. The reduction in the number of insulin receptors can also be produced in mice by treating them with gold thioglucose, which also makes them obese and insulin-resistant (Soll, Kahn, Neville, & Roth, 1975). In general, the higher the insulin level, the lower the number of receptors (Kahn, 1976).

Treatments that produce insulin deficiency have the opposite effect, causing an increase in the number of receptors (Goldfine, 1975; Soll, Kahn, Neville, & Roth, 1975). Correction of either the deficiency or overabundance of insulin returns the concentration of receptors to normal. The rate of decrease with high insulin is dependent on the concentration of insulin, with $10^{-7} M$ concentrations producing a 40% reduction in four hours. The return to normal is completed within 16 hours. Both the reduction and the return are dependent on protein synthesis (Kahn, 1976). There is one difference between these results and those with antigens: The reduction of receptors after antibody treatment was not blocked by inhibitors of protein synthesis (Raff, 1976).

Decreases in the number of hormone receptors after treatment with the hormones themselves have now been observed with growth hormone, thyrotropin-releasing hormone, progesterone, estrogen, and sometimes angiotensin (Lesniak & Roth, 1976). This relationship has not been found with prolactin, follicle-stimulating hormone, or luteinizing hormone, but the in vivo methodologies used with these hormones have been questioned (Lesniak & Roth, 1976).

One other report conflicting somewhat with the general pattern of higher hormone levels causing lower concentrations of their receptors showed that mice fed a diet high in carbohydrates did not lose receptors but rather sometimes gained more (Maugh, 1976). This diet produces short periods of high insulin immediately after eating, but a basal level somewhat lower than normal. From this it has been argued that it is only the basal level that is important for determining the number of receptors. The possibility remains, however, that the short periods of insulin also contributed to maintaining the number of receptors; at least, this is the result that would be most in line with the rest principle, because use followed by rest, not rest alone, is the requirement for increasing the strength of connections. This requirement might also explain the results with luteinizing hormone, in which a single in vivo injection caused an increase in the number of receptors (Lesniak & Roth, 1976). (It is clear that many of the workers in this field view the control of receptivity purely in terms of negative feedback [Kahn, 1976; Roth et al., 1977]. The one point in the rest principle that does not operate according to negative feedback is this requirement that a connection be used before resting in order to be strengthened.)

We return later to the hormone receptor reactions, but first let us examine systems in which the number of receptors is controlled by the level of putative neural transmitters. Mukherjee, Caron, and Lefkowitz (1975) found that beta-adrenergic agonists, isoproterenol and norepinephrine, produce a reduction in the beta-adrenergic receptors on frog erythrocytes. Kebabian, Zatz, Romero, and Axelrod (1975) found similar reductions in the receptors on pineal cells of rats using isoproterenol or prolonged exposure to dark to release norepinephrine. Fluctuations in the number of beta-adrenergic receptors in the pineal also occur naturally with circadian rhythms, indicating that the self-regulation of receptors also occurs physiologically. Consistent with these results, it had previously been found that repeated exposure to large concentrations of catecholamines caused subsensitivity in the pineal, but a decrease in norepinephrine produced supersensitivity (Deguchi & Axelrod, 1973).

Evidence suggesting that self-regulation of acetylcholine receptors may occur in muscles has been available for a long time (Kravitz, 1967). Axelsson and Thesleff (1959) showed that, after denervation, muscles developed receptors along their entire length, and it was later found that denervated muscles could be reinnervated at sites other than the original end plate (Frank et al., 1975). Denervated muscles first become subsensitive to cholinergic stimulation, while large amounts of transmitter are still being lost by the degenerating neurons and later become supersensitive when the acetylcholine is no longer present (Langer, 1975). Similarly, extraneous acetylcholine is known to produce desensitization of the motor end plate (Katz & Thesleff, 1957; Magavanik & Vyskočil, 1973), and the desensitization can be produced specifically in the muscle itself without involving the neurons (Lambert, Spannbauer & Parsons, 1977).

It now appears likely that these results are caused partially by changes in the number of acetylcholine receptors (Fambrough, 1974). After denervation the number of receptors increases about fifteen-fold (Almon, Andrew, & Appel, 1974; Appel, Roses, Almon, Andrew, Smith, McNamara, & Butterfield, 1975). The new receptors first appear scattered on the muscle but then gradually congregate into clusters; with time the clusters become larger but fewer in number (Ko, Anderson, & Cohen, 1977). Denervation also causes an increase in the turnover rate of acetylcholine receptors: Normally about 20% are lost per day, but after denervation 80% are lost per day (Berg & Hall, 1974).

One important question that remains to be answered for most systems is whether the changes in the number of receptor sites is determined by the degree to which the receptors themselves are filled with transmitter or by the rate at which the cellular response is produced. In the case of beta-adrenergic receptors, it has been found that although agonists reduce the number of sites, the antagonist, propranodol, not only does not cause a decrease but also blocks the decrease caused by agonists (Mukherjee & Lefkowitz, 1977). It has been suggested that these results show that receptor occupancy in this system is not sufficient for lowering the number of sites (Raff, 1976). In a very superficial way this is true because the antagonist does "occupy" the receptor. Occupancy by an antagonist is not, however, the same as occupancy by an agonist. First, it is clear that the conformation of the antagonist–receptor complex is different from that of the agonist–receptor complex. Second, it is likely that the conformation of the receptor itself is different when it is occupied by an antagonist than when it is filled with an agonist (Lester, 1977). Consequently, if the process responsible for the reduction of the number of receptors selectively attacks either the agonist-receptor-complex conformation or the receptor conformation when it contains agonists, the process probably would not attack receptors containing antagonists. Therefore, the results with antagonists do not show whether the loss of receptors is caused by occupancy or by the cellular response, because both the agonist-occupancy conformation and the response are probably eliminated by the antagonist.

In the acetylcholine receptors of muscles it appears that the presence of the nerve contributes to the supersensitivity. Artificially stimulating a muscle can repress the denervation changes, whereas inactivity alone can produce supersensitivity (Lømo & Rosenthal, 1972; Purves & Sakmann, 1974) and increase the number of receptors (Lavoie, Collier, & Tenenhouse, 1976; Pestronk,

Drachmann, & Griffin, 1976). Denervation, however, produces a greater increase in receptors than inactivity (Pestronk et al., 1976) and greater resistance to tetrodotoxin. Cangiano and Lutzember (1977) revived the suggestion that the degenerating nerve stump is partially responsible for supersensitivity by showing that innervated muscle fibers adjacent to denervated ones also have an increased resistance to tetrodotoxin. It is not possible to separate the effects of receptor occupancy from cellular responding, because the procedures used to produce inactivity block the release of transmitter.

Supersensitivity is found also after denervation or disuse of muscles supplied by adrenergic neurons (Langer, 1975). A trivial presynaptic factor contributing to supersensitivity is caused by the loss of uptake of agonist by the nerve, thus leaving more for the muscle. A postsynaptic factor may be caused by an increase in the number of receptors, as suggested by a decrease in the blocking ability of phenoxybenzamine, but conclusive evidence is not yet available.

Denervation supersensitivity, after initial subsensitivity, has also been demonstrated with the acetylcholine receptors of sweat glands (Reas & Trendelenberg, 1967) and salivary glands (Emmelin, 1964b). As with muscles, the subsensitivity is thought to be caused by a leakage of transmitter from the degenerating nerve. In glands this is accompanied by a profuse output. Supersensitivity may also be produced in glands by blocking the neural input. As with muscles, both denervation and disuse supersensitivity can be reversed or prevented by exercising the glands with, for instance, daily injections of pilocarpine. Also with acetylcholine receptors, but in the electric organ of some fish, it is well known that prolonged administration of the transmitter produces "pharmacological desensitization" (Changeux 1975). It has not yet been determined whether these changes are associated with alterations in the number of acetylcholine receptors.

Recently it was shown that prostaglandins cause a desensitization of the adenyl cyclase response in frog erythrocytes (Lefkowitz, Mullikin, Wood, Gore, & Mukherjee, 1977), and it was established that a decrease in the number of prostaglandin receptors was also produced. Guanine nucleotides are able to reverse the effect and rapidly restore the number of receptors.

In summary, there is a general rule for how the number of receptors on nonneuronal cells is regulated: The number decreases with overuse and increases with rest. This is in agreement with the rest principle and contrary to the use principle. The critical question then is whether the same rule applies as well to the receptors on neurons.

It had long been suspected that desensitization and denervation supersensitivity also occur in neurons. In 1949, Cannon and Rosenblueth suggested that supersensitivity is a widespread phenomenon occurring not only in muscles but also in the spinal cord and the brain. They reported indirect evidence that denervation of the superior cervical ganglion caused supersensitivity. This has been confirmed by others, but the indirectness of the evidence and conflicting data (see Sharpless, 1975) have prevented acceptance of the findings.

Disuse supersensitivity was first demonstrated in neurons by Beránek and Hník in 1959 and has since been replicated several times with additional controls (Goldfarb & Muller, 1971; Kozak & Westerman, 1961; Robbins & Nelson, 1970; Spencer & April, 1969). The general paradigm in these studies has been to stop the firing of certain afferent nerves stimulated by stretch receptors by removing the tension on the muscles containing these receptors. Later, the afferents are stimulated and the monosynaptic reflex produced is examined. It was found that the reflex became much stronger after disuse. The initial studies were subject to the possibility of confounding by the gamma efferent system, but the later studies have controlled for this (Spencer & April, 1969) and still found supersensitivity.

One interesting finding is that the supersensitivity is present only when the neurons that have been allowed to rest are tested. When other afferents having synapses on the same motoneurons are tested, the reflex is normal (Goldfarb & Muller, 1971; Robbins & Nelson, 1970). This is in agreement with the later finding that partial denervation of neurons does not affect the responsiveness to stimulation from the remaining inputs (Roper, 1976).

When slabs of cerebral cortex are undercut, the cells become overly susceptible to epileptic-like discharges after the general application of acetylcholine or electrical stimulation (see Sharpless, 1975). After repeated discharges the functioning returns to normal. Epileptic supersensitivity can be prevented by daily or even twice-weekly administration of subconvulsive electrical stimulation. Subsequent work with iontophoretic application of acetylcholine or L-glutamate showed, however, that fewer neurons than normal are excited in the isolated cortical slabs. The reason for this discrepancy is not yet clear.

One explanation for the increased epileptic-like susceptibility after the general application of acetylcholine is that the concentration of acetylcholinesterase is reduced in isolated cortical slabs. A parallel complication is found in denervation supersensitivity of muscles. Both denervation and axoplasmic transport blockage, which produce supersensitivity, result in substantial reductions in the total level of acetylcholinesterase activity (Inestrosa, Ramírez, & Fernandez, 1977), although inactivity alone does not affect the amount of the enzyme at the end plate (Steinbach, 1974). Denervation also causes the enzyme to be found in the plasma. The release and loss of enzyme may be the result of the loss of cellular contact between the nerve and muscle (Inestrosa et al. 1977). The reduced enzyme activity after denervation could be partially responsible for the greater effect of this treatment than inactivity (Cangiano and Lutzemberger, 1977) and perhaps also for the longer duration that acetylcholine channels remain open in denervated than in normal muscle fibers (Neher & Sakmann, 1976).

The first generally accepted demonstration of denervation supersensitivity in neurons was by Kuffler, Dennis, and Harris (1971), who found an increased chemosensitivity in the parasympathetic ganglion cells of the frog heart after denervation. As with supersensitivity in muscles, the increased responsiveness was found in extrasynaptic areas, thus suggesting the development of new receptors. Roper (1976) studied the acetylcholine sensitivity of the parasympathetic ganglion neurons of the mud puppy after partial denervation, both in vivo and in vitro. Supersensitivity to acetylcholine was found in both cases, though it developed more slowly in vivo.

Denervation is more difficult to study in the central nervous system, but there are various ways of either producing selective lesions or otherwise reducing the amount of transmitter being received. The first studies produced lesions of the dopamine pathways with the administration of 6-hydroxydopamine to one hemisphere of the brain. Subsequently, apomorphine, a dopamine agonist, was given, and the animals were found to turn in circles. The rotating behavior indicated that the previously lesioned hemisphere was now supersensitive to the agonist (Ungerstedt, 1971a, 1971b). Supersensitivity to microinjections of dopamine was subsequently shown in 6-hydroxydopamine pretreated cats (Feltz & DeChamplain, 1972). An effect of dopamine on the response in caudate nucleus cells to nigral stimulation was found in the lesioned cats but not in controls. Similarly, an effect from dopamine on the response to amino acid-induced discharge in the caudate was found in all of the lesioned cats but in only 43% of the normal ones. In another study (Siggins, Hoffer, & Ungerstedt, 1974), the response of striatal cells to iontophoretic applications of dopamine and apomorphine was found to be enhanced in lesioned animals. Stereotypic behavioral responses to subthreshold doses of apomorphine are also produced by the lesion.

It has now been shown that the denervation supersensitivity of dopamine receptors is associated with an increase in the number of receptor sites (Creese, Burt, & Snyder, 1977). The percentage of increase ranged from about 20 to 120%. The increase in receptor sites was related to the increase in rotational behavior after apomorphine. The behavioral changes, however, were larger than would be expected from the increase in the number of receptors, suggesting that other factors also were helping to enhance the rotation. The affinity of the individual receptors was not changed.

Supersensitivity to dopaminergic agonists can be produced in several other ways. Treatment with the dopamine antagonist haloperidol produces behavioral supersensitivity (Gianutsos, Drawbaugh, Hynes, & Lal, 1974), although the effect is seen more clearly in the dopamine receptors implicated in motor behavior than in those affecting thermoregulation (Costentin, Protais, & Schwartz, 1975). Even a single injection of haloperidol or another neuroleptic, teflutixol, can produce supersensitivity (Hyttel & Nielsen, 1976). Initially a decrease in sterotypic gnawing behavior is produced, apparently by the blockade of the receptors. This is followed by an increase in the amount of gnawing produced by apomorphine. Dopamine synthesis is increased during the initial subsensitivity phase but decreased during the supersensitivity phase (Hyttel, 1975). Apparently this relationship exists because receptor blockade inhibits a negative-feedback mechanism (such as the unusual dendritic interaction with GABA interneurons [Dismukes, 1977] that are discussed later), thus allowing increased firing of the dopamine neurons and increased dopamine synthesis. During supersensitivity, the negative-feedback system is overly active and suppresses firing and synthesis of the dopamine. Hyttel and Nielsen (1976) were able to show that supersensitivity produced by neuroleptics such as haloperidol is caused by an increase of some kind in the dopamine receptor sensitivity. Burt, Creese, and Snyder (1977) then demonstrated that the supersensitivity 5 days after the end of chronic haloperidol administration was associated with a 20–25% increase in the number of receptors. The individual receptors showed no significant change in their affinity. For fluphenazine, another neuroleptic, no data were reported for the individual affinities, but the total increase in binding was similar to that with haloperidol, suggesting that the number of receptors probably increased to a similar extent. Muller and Seeman (1977) showed that chronic haloperidol has a rather specific effect on dopamine receptors. The binding of dopaminergic antagonist and agonist increased 34 and 77% in the striatum and 45 and 55% in the mesolimbic area. The binding of serotonin, alpha-adrenergic agonist, and naloxone was, in general, not significantly increased; the only exceptions were serotonin in the striatum and alpha-adrenergic agonist in the cortex, which increased 20 and 13% respectively.

A third method for producing behavioral supersensitivity to dopaminergic agonists is chronic administration of reserpine, which depletes the brain of the transmitter (Moore & Thornburg, 1975; Tarsy & Baldessarini, 1974; Von Voigtlander, Losey, & Triezenberg, 1975). This is associated with a 20% increase in the binding of (^3H)haloperidol, probably reflecting a similar increase in the number of receptors.

The fourth method for producing dopaminergic supersensitivity is the administration of inhibitors of the synthesis of dopamine, alpha-methyltyrosine (Annunziato & Moore, 1977; Dominic & Moore, 1969) or alpha-methylparatyrosine (Costentin et al., 1977). This method avoids the problem of residential antagonist found with the use of neuroleptics and the problem of the initial increase in the release of transmitter found after lesioning or the administration of reserpine. With the other methods, supersensitivity is not seen until about 2 days after the treatment. Administration of alpha-methylparatyrosine, however, enhanced climbing behavior from dopamine agonists at only 2 hours. Because the reduction in dopamine levels itself was not immediate but just beginning at 2 hours, it is likely that the development of supersensitivity actually requires much less than 2 hours to begin. The supersensitivity in this case could be blocked by cycloheximide and/or anisomycin, demonstrating that it was dependent on protein synthesis.

In addition to acetylcholine and dopamine, denervation supersensitivity has now been found for beta-adrenergic receptors in neurons (Kendall, Wolfe,

Sporn, Poulos, & Molinoff, 1977; Sporn et al., 1976). The denervation procedure used was the same as that in the initial dopamine studies (i.e., the administration of 6-hydroxydopamine, which destroys norepinephrine as well as
dopamine neurons). The concentration of beta-adrenergic receptors in the cerebral cortex was then examined. In the study by Sporn et al., using adult rats, the
mean number of these receptors was increased by 31%. The affinity of the
individual receptors was not changed significantly.

Kendall et al. (1977) studied the effects of 6-hydroxydopamine lesions on the
development of beta-adrenergic receptors in rats, giving the compound systemically on the first to fourth days after birth, when the blood brain barrier has not
yet developed. Normally, rats show an increase in the density of beta-adrenergic
receptors during the first weeks after birth. The lesioned rats had a similar time
course for the development of the receptors, but at all time points, from 6 to 45
days, they had 45 to 75% more receptors than the controls.

These rest-induced increases in norepinephrine, dopamine, and probably
acetylcholine receptors on neurons were included in my review article on the
physiological evidence for the rest principle (Sinclair, 1978). GABA can now be
added to the list (Waddington & Cross, 1978). Kainic acid was used to destroy
neurons releasing GABA. This caused a subsequent behavioral supersensitivity
to a drug (muscimal) that activates GABA receptors. It also caused an increased
binding of radioactive GABA, which, together with no change in the dissociation
constant, indicated that the number of GABA receptors had increased.

It is possible that the increase in receptors on neurons after denervation has
already been seen with an electron microscope. Gulley, Wenthold, and Neises
(1977) examined the ultrastructure change in the anteroventral nucleus neurons
after denervation by cochlear ablation. There are particular particles that normally are found mostly in synaptic areas, and it is tempting to equate these
particles with receptors. Denervation caused a large increase in the number of
these particles outside the synaptic areas, reminiscent of the spread of receptors.
At the shortest interval examined, 12 hours after the operation, they had increased by 147%. The number of particles continued increasing for 6 days. When
the neurons were reinnervated, the number then declined. There is, of course, no
proof yet that these particles are in fact receptors.

Desensitization of neurons by large concentrations of transmitter is also well
established. Curtis and Ryall (1966) showed that acetylcholine could desensitize
Renshaw cells in the spinal column, in a way similar to that seen at the
neuromuscular junction. In the central nervous system, desensitization of the
inhibitory effects of dopamine has been demonstrated (York, 1970). Desensitization of the dominergic and adrenergic receptors controlling thermoregulation also
has been reported (Chiel, Yehuda, & Wurtman, 1974; Costentin et al., 1975).
Reduced sensitivity is shown by the presynaptic alpha-adrenergic receptors after
administration of norepinephrine (Langer & Dubocovich, 1977). Pretreatment
with d-amphetamine produced a subsensitivity to norepinephrine but not to

dopamine, as measured by the cyclic AMP response (Martres, Baudry, & Schwartz, 1975). Similarly, MAO inhibition, which increases the norepinephrine level, reduced the reactivity of the cyclic AMP system to norepinephrine (Vatulani et al., 1976).

At present there is little information concerning the mechanism responsible for desensitization. Burt et al. (1977) examined the binding of haloperidol in the brains of five rats pretreated with amphetamine and found no significant change, but the negative result has little bearing on desensitization, because amphetamine does not reduce the responsiveness of dopaminergic receptors. On the other hand, in the same study the increases in binding produced by 3 weeks of pretreatment with haloperidol decreased as a function of the number of drug-free days. Significant increases of 24–25% were found after 5 drug-free days. After 12 days these had declined to 13–18%, and after 17 days without haloperidol only nonsignificant increases of 0–8% were found. So it appears that at least the relative desensitization related to the loss of supersensitivity may be associated with a decrease in the number of receptor sites. No data were reported, however, for the affinity of the individual receptors in the groups with longer drug-free periods. Consequently, the possibility cannot be eliminated that, although the initial increase in binding was caused by an increase in the number of receptors, the subsequent return of binding to approximately normal was caused by a decrease in affinity.

The evidence concerning the effects of prolonged opiate agonists on the number of opiate receptors is still ambiguous. One report stated that the number of receptor sites was not changed 72–84 hours after implantation of morphine pellets, but at five of the six test concentrations the implanted animals showed less narcotic binding than the controls, a tendency that was not significant perhaps because of the small number of animals (Klee & Streaty, 1974). Pert, Pasternak, and Snyder (1973) showed that implantation of opiate antagonists produces large rapid increases in the number of opiate receptors. This appears to be similar to the increases in dopamine receptors caused by blocking agents (i.e., the antagonists block opiate receptors and the resulting rest causes the number of receptors to increase). They also found, however, that opiate agonists caused small increases in receptors, in contradiction to the tendency noted in the study by Klee and Streaty. The sensitivity of opiate-receptor reactivity to sodium concentrations may have introduced complications and may be partially responsible for the discrepancy.

There are various hypotheses as to what happens to "lost" receptors after persistent high concentrations of transmitter are experienced (Kolata, 1977). One possibility is that the receptors containing transmitter are broken down. Consistent with this idea, hormone-receptor complexes have now been found in lysosomes. It also has been found that radioactive calcitonin remains in the bone after it has caused a reduction in the number of its receptors.

Another possibility is that receptors exist in a densitized conformation, in which the transmitter is tightly bound but the cellular response is not produced (Lefkowitz et al., 1977; Lester, 1977). Lefkowitz et al. have proposed the following model for the removal of functional prostaglandin receptor:

$$H + R \rightleftharpoons HR$$
$$\updownarrow \qquad \updownarrow$$
$$H + R' \rightleftharpoons HR'$$

where H is hormone, R is the normal receptor with a low affinity, and R' is a desensitized receptor with a high affinity. The dissociation of HR to $H + R$ is therefore faster than that of HR' to $H + R'$. It is also assumed that interactions between the HR complex and adenylate cyclase, producing cyclic AMP and the cellular response, cause the receptor to take on the desensitized conformation R' and that this reaction normally is favored over the reverse reaction converting HR' to HR. Thus the number of open receptors is reduced after large amounts of hormone because many of the receptors are still filled.

Lester's model for the acetylcholine receptor is somewhat similar. In his model, a third receptor conformation appears, a resting state in which the receptor binds best to antagonists. Receptors in the high affinity desensitized conformation are then assumed to change preferentially to the resting conformation.

These models work well for explaining the reduction in the number of functional receptors with desensitization, and they also can explain why denervation or disuse causes an increase in the number of functional receptors; however, they do not explain why disuse causes receptors to appear in new locations nor why protein synthesis is required to increase the number of receptors. This does not mean that they are wrong but merely incomplete, and other processes also must be involved in the self-regulation of receptors.

In summary, the number of receptors on neurons, as well as on nonneuronal cells, is generally regulated in accordance with the rest principle. This is illustrated in Fig. 6.1.

Changing the number of receptors is just one way in which postsynaptic receptivity could be varied in accordance with the rest principle. Another such process, working on a shorter time scale, involves "negative cooperativity." Cooperativity is present when the binding of one receptor to its transmitter affects the affinity of other receptors. If the affinity increases with increasing concentrations of transmitter, "positive cooperativity" is present. If the filling of one receptor makes it harder for the others to capture a transmitter molecule, then negative cooperativity is said to occur. Negative cooperativity is frequently found with hormones and neural transmitters; positive cooperativity is very rare in these systems, but lack of cooperativity is also common.

Negative cooperativity has been clearly established for the insulin receptor (DeMeyts, Bianco, & Roth, 1976; DeMeyts & Roth, 1975; DeMeyts, Roth,

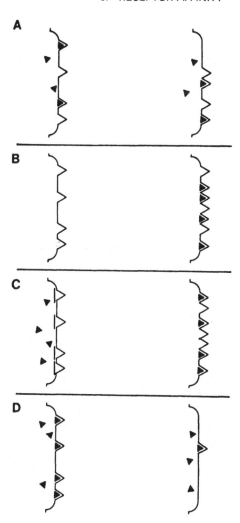

FIG. 6.1. Summary of how the number of postsynaptic receptors for transmitter (▲) is controlled. A. With moderate amounts of transmitter (left), the number of receptors remains about the same (right), despite the removal of some receptors and the development of some new ones. B. Absence of transmitter (left) causes an increase in the number of receptors (right) and the potential for an exaggerated response (i.e., supersensitivity) when transmitter returns (Four receptors are filled in contrast to only two in A.). C. Blocking receptors (left) also causes an increase in the number of receptors and supersensitivity (right). D. Excessive amounts of transmitter (left) cause a reduction in the number of receptors and subsensitivity (right).

Neville, Gavin, & Lesniak, 1973; Freychet, Rosselin, Rancon, Foucereau, & Broer, 1974; Ginsberg, Cohen, & Kahn, 1976; Soll, Kahn, & Neville, 1975). High levels of insulin decrease the affinity of the remaining unfilled receptors about tenfold, perhaps as a result of the observed decrease in the size of the receptors (Ginsberg et al., 1976).

Negative cooperativity has now been found with thyroid-stimulating hormone receptors in the thyroid (Tate, Holmes, Kohn, & Winard, 1975; Verrier, Fayet, & Lisitzky, 1974); and thyroid-releasing factor receptors in the pituitary (Grant, Vale, & Guillemin, 1973). Lack of cooperativity is shown by the receptors for luteinizing hormone, angiotensin, and growth hormone (Kahn, 1976; Lesniak & Roth, 1976). Vasopressin is the only hormone known to produce positive cooperativity among its receptors (Bockaert, Roy, Rajerison, & Jard , 1973; Jard, Roy, Barth, Rajerison, & Bockaert, 1975).

With neural transmitters, negative cooperativity has been found for the beta-adrenergic receptors in frog erythrocytes (Limbird, DeMeyts, & Lefkowitz, 1975; Mukherjee, Caron, Coverstone, & Lefkowitz, 1975), but lack of cooperativity was reported with turkey erythrocytes (Aurbach, Fedak, Wood-ward, Palmer, Hauser, & Troxer, 1974; Brown, Hauser, Troxler, & Aurbach, 1976). Lack of cooperativity (Cohen & Changeux, 1975; Klett, Fulpuis, Cooper, Smith, Reich, & Possani, 1973) and both positive and negative cooperativity (Eldefrawi & Eldefrawi, 1973; Eldefrawi, Eldefrawi, Seifert, & O'Brian, 1972; Lester, 1977) have been reported for the electric-organ cholinergic receptors.

The supersensitivity in denervated muscles may be caused partly by changes in affinity as well as by the fifteen-fold increase in the number of receptors (Almon et al., 1974; Appel et al., 1975). In normal muscles the acetylcholine receptors have an affinity of $10^8 \, l$/mol. Treatment with detergent raises their affinity to $10^9 \, l$/mol. In denervated muscles, however, the affinity is already $10^9 \, l$/mol, and detergent treatment causes no change. Appel et al. concluded that the increase was not caused by a change in the primary conformation of the receptor but by a different molecular interaction of the receptor with its environment. That a conformational change does occur in situ is suggested by the finding that a globulin from patients with *Myasthenia gravis* binds to denervated muscle acetylcholine receptors but not to the receptors in normal muscles.

Over short periods of time (i.e., less than about a minute), it is likely that positive cooperativity is shown in the binding of acetylcholine by muscle receptors and that this factor dominates in determining the responsiveness of the muscle. Over longer periods of time, however, negative-feedback factors, such as an increase in the number of desensitized receptors, play a more important role than positive cooperativity (Lester, 1977). The advantages of such an arrangement are discussed in the section on presynaptic factors.

In neurons there is little evidence for the occurrence of cooperativity. In peripheral neurons, the binding of nerve-growth factor shows negative cooperativity (Frazier, Boyd, & Bradshaw, 1974). The increased number of beta-adrenergic receptors in the cerebral cortex after 6-hydroxydopamine lesions does not show either positive or negative cooperativity (Sporn et al., 1976). In other studies with neurons, data on cooperativity have not been reported.

It generally has been found that denervation and disuse do not affect the affinity of individual receptors in neurons. Serotonin, however, seems to be an exception. Reduced serotonin levels produce supersensitivity, as occurs with other transmitters. The supersensitivity with serotonin seems to be caused by an increased receptor affinity rather than by an increase in the number of receptors (Trulson & Jacobs, 1978; Wirz-Justice, Krauchi, Lichtsteiner, & Feer, 1978).

There is evidence suggesting that ''second-messenger'' systems play an intermediate role between the filling of receptors with agonists and the production of a cellular response. In many cases this second-messenger system seems to involve the conversion of ATP into cyclic AMP by specific adenylate cyclases (Nathanson, 1977). There are two ways in which the cyclic AMP response is of interest here. First, it can be used as an index of postsynaptic receptivity and, as such, gives additional evidence for the existence of supersensitivity and desensitization. Second, there now are suggestions that the cyclic AMP system itself may contribute to these effects and not merely reflect changes in the number or affinity of receptors.

Numerous studies have shown that denervation with 6-hydroxydopamine, treatment with reserpine, and other procedures reducing occupancy of norepinephrine receptors increase cyclic AMP accumulation produced by norepinephrine or isoproterenol (Dismukes & Daly, 1975; Huang & Daly, 1974; Huang, Ho, & Daly, 1973; Kalisker, Rutledge, & Perkins, 1973; Kendall et al., 1977; Palmer, 1972; Palmer, Sulser, & Robinson, 1973; Sporn et al., 1976; Strada, Uzunov, & Weiss, 1971; Vetulani et al., 1976; Williams & Pirch, 1974). For dopamine-stimulated adenylate cyclase, the data are not so unanimous, but the majority of the reports (Gnegy, Uzunov, & Costa, 1977; Mishra, Gardner, Katzman, & Makman, 1974; Nathanson, 1977) show increases in cyclic AMP accumulation in animals given chronic treatments reducing the filling of receptors with dopamine, whereas the others show no change (Krueger, Forn, Walters, Roth, & Greengard, 1976; Von Voigtlander et al., 1973).

Treatments that produce long-term increases in norepinephrine reduce the cyclic AMP response caused by beta-adrenergic agonists in erythrocytes (Mickey, Tate, & Lefkowitz, 1975; Mukherjee, Caron, & Lefkowitz, 1975) and in the central nervous system (Martres et al., 1975; Vetulani et al., 1976).

In the study by Sporn et al. (1976), the number of receptors increased only 31% in the 6-hydroxydopamine lesioned rats, whereas the maximal accumulation of cyclic AMP increased by 80%. Similarly, the behavioral supersensitivity to dopaminergic agonists after haloperidol pretreatment was greater than the increase in the number of receptors (Burt et al., 1977). The reason for these discrepancies could be partially that the cyclic AMP system also becomes more reactive and that supersensitivity is the combined result of both more receptors and a more active second messenger system, as has been suggested (Gnegy et al., 1977; Nathanson, 1977; Vetulani et al, 1976). Conversely, it has been hypothesized by Nathanson, 1977 that: "chronic overstimulation of adenylate cyclase receptors may lead to a decrease synthesis and/or activity of the enzyme [p. 196]."

One way in which the cyclic AMP system could contribute to supersensitivity was discovered by Gnegy, Uzunov, and Costa (1976). Bound to the membrane of the postsynaptic neuron is a calcium (Ca^{2+}) binding protein that activates adenylate cyclase. They now have found that the amount of this activator increases after haloperidol or (+)-butochamol pretreatments that induce supersensitivity (Gnegy et al., 1977). Desensitization, on the other hand, might be partially caused by a removal of this activator from the membrane. Cyclic AMP causes phosphorylation of the binding site of the protein, releasing it into the cytosol. Therefore, large amounts of dopamine present for a long period of time could, through the persistent production of cyclic AMP, reduce the amount of bound activator. This would then reduce the sensitivity of the dopamine adenylate cyclase.

Interestingly, the discrepancy between the increase in the number of receptors and the increase in the cyclic AMP response was not seen in developing rats (Kendall et al., 1977). The procedures used were similar to those employed by Sporn et al. (1976) in adult rats; indeed, both studies come from the same laboratory. The only difference was that 6-hydroxydopamine was now given systemically to newborn rats instead of being given intraventricularly to adult rats. The increase in receptor sites was somewhat greater than in animals lesioned as adults (45–75% versus 31%), whereas the increase in the maximal accumulation of cyclic AMP was somewhat smaller (40–65% versus 80%). The greater increase in receptors may be the result of a greater reduction of norepinephrine stores in the animals treated just after birth. The smaller increase in cyclic AMP response may be partly a reflection of a slight increase in the basal levels of cyclic AMP accumulation found in rats lesioned as adults. It also suggests that supersensitivity in the cyclic AMP system may require that the system be activated before being allowed to rest.

Considering the difficulties involved in studies such as these and the little we know about confounding variables, it would be wise to use caution when considering the discrepancies between the changes in the number of receptors and the cyclic AMP system and the differences between studies. The suggestion that the cyclic AMP system may contribute to supersensitivity and desensitization, although reasonable, is based on a relatively weak empirical foundation, and much more work needs to be done before definite conclusions can be made. The major problem involves the second-messenger hypothesis. In at least one system, the dopamine synapses of the cervical ganglion neurons, there is relatively good evidence that the cyclic AMP produced when dopamine is received does not act as a second messenger for the production of postsynaptic electrical potentials. Dopamine here causes an inhibitory postsynaptic potential, but direct injection of cyclic AMP does not (Kobayashi, Hashiguchi, & Ushiyama, 1978). Instead, it produces a facilitation of the slow excitatory postsynaptic potentials produced by muscarinic acetylcholine synapses on the same postsynaptic neurons. As a result, these cells become easier to fire for long periods of time after the dopamine neurons have fired onto them or after cyclic AMP has been experimentally administered. These "dopamine junctions" and their possible roles are discussed in detail in Chapter 10.

In summary, although different mechanisms may contribute to regulation of the responsiveness of postsynaptic neurons, all the known or postulated mechanisms act in such a way that responsiveness changes in accordance with the rest principle, decreasing with overuse and increasing with rest. No mechanism has been identified that would control responsiveness in the way required by the use principle.

So far we have been concerned with changes in the receptivity of the post-synaptic neuron. Although it seems likely that these changes are important in learning, we cannot conclude that other factors do not play a role also. Changes in presynaptic functioning are considered first.

Contrary to the classical view, it now seems clear that the amount of transmitter released with each action potential is not fixed. This conclusion was reached in a review by Stjärne in 1975 and has since been confirmed in a large number of studies. It is the changes in these quanta secreted per nerve impulse that have been the focus of interest for presynaptic studies of plasticity. In general, for very short periods of time the release is governed by positive feedback, but negative feedback predominates on intermediate and long-term time scales (Fig. 6.2).

Although there are some conflicting data with different systems (Stjärne, 1975), in general, when several impulses per second arrive at the presynaptic terminal, the amount of transmitter released per impulse increases with the input frequency, so that much larger amounts are released per stimulation at 10 Hz than at 1 Hz (Stjärne & Brundin, 1977b). This relationship is thought to be caused by the electrical properties of the membranes. At very high frequencies, the relationship breaks down and the quanta released per impulse at 30 Hz is less than at 10 Hz. The limiting factor does not seem to be in the capacity of the axon to carry such high rates of stimulation but rather in the secretory process itself: If release in general is inhibited, the quanta secreted per impulse at 30 Hz become greater than at 10 Hz.

Negative feedback has been studied most thoroughly in norepinephrine synapses. Located on the presynaptic neuron are alpha-adrenergic receptors, or "alpha$_2$-adrenergic receptors" according to the classification by Berthelson and Pettinger (1977). These sense the norepinephrine concentration in their vicinity and suppress the subsequent quanta per impulse released accordingly (Enero, Langer, Rothlin, & Stefano, 1972; Langer and Dubocovich, 1977; Starke, 1972; Stjärne, 1975; Stjärne & Brundin, 1977a, 1977b; Wennmalm, 1971). There are compounds capable of blocking specifically the alpha-adrenergic receptors and not the beta-adrenergic receptors; such compounds increase the amount of norepinephrine secreted per impulse. The supersensitivity produced by cocaine, for instance, is believed to occur because of its blocking of alpha-adrenergic receptors (Langer, 1975). Similarly, at an early stage after denervation the presynaptic alpha-adrenergic receptors become subsensitive, and increased quanta of transmitter are released with each stimulation of the nerve (Langer and Dubocovich, 1977).

A second negative feedback system in adrenergic synapses involves prostaglandin E_2 (Hedqvist, 1969; Stjärne & Brundin, 1977a, 1977b). The release of norepinephrine is associated with the local release of prostaglandin E_2, which then also causes an inhibition of subsequent norepinephrine output. Inhibitors of prostaglandin production, consequently, cause an increase in the amount of transmitter released per impulse (Stjärne & Brundin, 1977b). A third influence on norepinephrine release has now been demonstrated: a facilitory, rather than inhibitory, action from beta-adrenergic agonists (Stjärne & Brundin, 1976). The

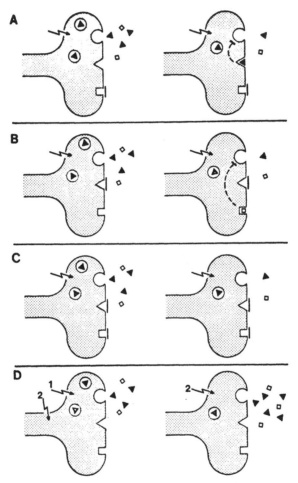

FIG. 6.2.   Factors affecting the release of transmitter (▲). A. Negative-feedback control by presynaptic receptors for the transmitter, even when the receptors for the controlling substance (□), such as prostaglandin, are blocked. B. Negative-feedback control by controlling substance, even when the receptors for the transmitter are blocked. C. Negative-feedback control by unidentified "fatigue factor," even when both types of receptors are blocked. D. Positive feedback: The first action potential potentiates release by a second coming shortly after it. This effect lasts for only a few milliseconds. The negative-feedback factors last much longer.

evidence at present suggests that all three of these factors work relatively independently (Stjärne & Brundin, 1977a).

In cholinergic synapses multiple stimuli generally produce a greater response per impulse than single stimuli, but the evidence so far suggests that this is not due to an increase in the quantal release of transmitter, as was usually found with adrenergic synapses. Instead, the amount of transmitter per stimulus stays roughly constant in some systems and decreases in others during short trains of stimulation (Stjärne, 1975). A negative-feedback system involving muscarinic receptors appears to function somewhat as does the alpha-adrenergic feedback in some cholinergic synapses (Polak, 1971).

Beyond the negative feedback controlled by alpha-adrenergic, prostaglandin E_2, and muscarinic receptors, there are additional factors that have been lumped together as "fatigue." Fatigue still can be seen after the alpha-adrenergic receptors are blocked and the production of prostaglandin is inhibited (Stjärne & Brundin, 1977b). With cholinergic synapses it also has been found that the response to stimulation is reduced if it is preceded by another stimulation and a suitable time interval separates the two. This can be seen with nicotinic junctions for which there is no evidence of transmitter negative feedback. The mechanisms responsible for secretory fatigue are not yet known. Studies have indicated that cyclic AMP also acts as a regulator factor in transmitter release and that it plays a greater role in fatigued neurons (Miyamoto & Breckenridge, 1974; Wilson, 1974). Other factors suggested include a depletion of available transmitter, a failure to synthesize transmitter fast enough, failure to recapture and reuse it, or a failure to mobilize the existing stores of transmitter (Stjärne, 1975).

Little is known about presynaptic feedback with transmitters other than norepinephrine and acetylcholine. A type of negative feedback is present, however, in the dopamine-secreting neurons in the substantia nigra. Local application of dopamine reduces the unit activity of these cells (Aghajanian & Bunney, 1973), whereas application of dopamine-receptor blocking agents increases activity (Bunney, Walters, Roth, & Aghajanian, 1973). It has now been suggested by Iversen (see Dismukes, 1977) that the negative feedback involves an unusual interaction with GABA-releasing interneurons also in the area. Dopamine is thought to be released from the dendrites, as well as by the distant terminals of the axons. The dendritically released dopamine could then stimulate the interneurons, causing GABA to be released, which would inhibit further firing of the dopamine-releasing neurons.

Although use may decrease the amount of norepinephrine or acetylcholine released per nerve impulse by various means, disuse of a nerve can increase the quanta secreted per stimulation. This was initially found for the splenic nerve releasing norepinephrine (Brown, Dearnaley, & Geffen, 1967) and subsequently for the cholinergic soleus neuromuscular junction (Robbins & Fischbach, 1971).

Although the increase in transmitter release occurs with relatively long periods of disuse, the data considered so far showing decreases in release have dealt with very short or intermediate time periods. There is, however, some evidence that long-term decreases in the release of transmitter can occur. Much of this evidence has come from studies of the reinnervation of muscles. In some systems, an organ reinnervated by neurons from two different sources will maintain functional synapses with both, but in some other systems competition occurs, and one set of synapses becomes nonfunctional (see Lømo, 1978; Mark, 1978). The loss of function has been shown in some cases to be caused by a drastic decrease in the amount of transmitter released per action potential (Grinnell, Rheuben, & Letinsky, 1977; Yip & Dennis, 1976). Mark (1978) has suggested that the repression may be caused by the production of a defect in the ion channel that in normal neurons allows calcium to enter the presynaptic nerve ending during the action potential. Calcium seems to be required universally for the release of transmitters (Rubin, 1970), and the failure of the calcium channel could prevent secretion, creating a "silent synapse."

Reduced transmitter release may be important in some neuronal systems for the production of habituation. The sea slug, *Aplysia*, usually withdraws its gills after stimulation, but this defensive reaction habituates after repeated stimulations. Because of the simple anatomy of the nervous system in *Aplysia* and the large size of some of the individual neurons, it has been possible to locate the specific synapses between the sensory input and the motor output governing this response. During habituation, the amount of transmitter released at these synapses per impulse decreased progressively until no detectable quantities were secreted. The synapses then remained silent for long periods of time. After prolonged use the synapses were nonfunctional for several weeks, and it is possible that they never would have recovered completely. It is not yet known if this extremely long debilitation is caused by failure to release transmitter (Castellucci, Carew, & Kandel, 1979; Mark, 1978).

It seems to be accepted that a loss of function can occur in the synapses in some systems. There is disagreement, however, as to whether the loss is caused by a reduction in the quantal release of transmitter or by a withdrawal of synaptic endings. Although degeneration appears to have been eliminated by electron microscopy experiments (Mark, 1978), some recent findings suggest that active withdrawal of synapses may indeed occur (Lømo, 1978). As is the case with many polemic arguments, it seems likely that both sides are right and that both repression of presynaptic output and withdrawal of synapses take place, perhaps in different systems or at different stages within a single system. Of more importance here is the fact that all current evidence suggests that the loss of functional synapses, by whatever means, occurs in a negative-feedback manner. The synapse in *Aplysia* became silent when it was used very frequently for long periods of time. The loss of presynaptic functioning in the reinnervation studies occurred when a single muscle fiber was innervated by two different neurons (Grinnell, et al., 1977), perhaps in this case because the muscle fiber was being excited too frequently.

In summary, with the exception of one mechanism with a very short time course, the release of transmitter is regulated in accordance with the rest principle. As a result of several mechanisms, the amount of transmitter released per action potential decreases with continual use and increases with rest. This is illustrated in Fig. 6.2.

The one possibility remaining to be discussed for changing the strength of the connections between neurons is the growth and retreating of neuronal processes and the formation and breaking of synapses. That such events can occur in mature animals is shown by lesion and denervation studies. Furthermore, the evidence from these studies suggests that the mechanisms operate in accordance with the rest principle, with new growth and new synapses forming on denervated targets.

During development, receptors for acetylcholine appear on muscle fibers after differentiation (Patrick, Heinemann, Lindstrom, Schubert, & Steinbach, 1972). Initially these are spread uniformly over the surface of the fibers, but later they cluster together into acetylcholine "hot spots" where the number of receptors is similar to that at the neuromuscular junctions (Sytkowski, Vogel, & Nirenberg, 1973). It has been suggested that these patches of receptors might be targets for growing nerve fibers.

As mentioned earlier, a similar sequence of events occurs in denervated muscles, first with new receptors appearing uniformly over the surface and then with clusters developing (Ko et al., 1977). Normally an innervated muscle rejects additional innervation, but a denervated fiber will accept it (Frank et al., 1975). Thus it appears that the clusters of receptors after denervation may also act as targets for neurons, as has been suggested repeatedly before.

We have seen that inactivity produced by depletion of the transmitter, blocking of the receptors, inhibition of release, or inhibition of the production of the transmitter also can produce supersensitivity in muscles and nerves. It therefore is possible that a neuron not receiving an adequate amount of transmitter, or blocked from producing its usual response to the transmitter (e.g., excitatory or inhibitory postsynaptic potentials), may develop new synaptic patches and take new innervation from neurons releasing that transmitter.

There is now clear evidence that denervation of neurons stimulates growth of other neurons and the development of new synapses. After lesions of axonal pathways of mature rats, surviving nerve terminals can proliferate and innervate the synaptic sites vacated by the degenerating axons (Raisman, 1977). Similarly, after cutting the input to the superior cervical ganglion, growth occurs at the stump and reinnervates the cells (Purves, 1976). If a nearby pathway also is cut and positioned near the ganglion, axons grow from both stumps, and both innervate the cells, with the normal input axons making more synapses. Such growth could have been stimulated by the cutting of the pathways. Courtney and Roper (1976) found, however, that crushing the right preganglion nerve to the frog cardiac ganglion produced sprouting in the intact left preganglion nerves, which then proceeded to reinnervate the right ganglion. Similarly, parasympathetic ganglion cells deprived of their normal input sprout and form synapses on each other, a form of innervation that normally does not occur (Sargent & Dennis,

1977). Such sprouting has now been found according to Courtney and Roper (1976) "in the central nervous system, the autonomic nervous system and peripheral nervous system and seems to be a characteristic response of nervous tissue to partial denervation." In the adult rat, sprouting normally takes 4 days; but if a preliminary lesion is made, the second lesion takes only 2 days to make sprouting occur (Scheff, Bernardo, & Cotman, 1977).

It is unclear what instigates the growth. It is possible that the stimulus comes from the degenerating neurons. In this case it would not occur in normal situations, and separate explanations would have to be made for the growth that occurs in development. Purves (1976) suggested that a neuron has a normal quota of synapses to make. If these are lost, it is stimulated to produce more. If it cannot do so, it loses its own innervation. If it is induced to make more than its quota, the surplus synapses often can be surplanted by synapses from neurons that have not reached their quota. On the other hand, neurons can be stimulated to make more than their quota of synapses by the presence of denervated cells. It seems necessary to postulate some humoral influence, such as nerve-growth factor, at least in the cases where the sprouting axons have not been directly affected by the lesion; somehow, the intact right preganglion neurons must find out that the left one has been crushed and that the left ganglion is denervated. Finally, it has been found that afferents deprived of their normal targets appear to induce abnormal dendritic growth in the pyramidal cells of the dentate gyrus, thus providing themselves with targets (Laurberg & Hjorth- Simonsen, 1977). Thus it seems that growth can occur to compensate for a lack of synaptic outputs, a lack of innervation, or a lack of targets. There are, however, various interpretations for these findings, and the only clear conclusion that can be made now is that denervation somehow stimulates growth and reinnervation.

The stimulation of axonal growth to denervated neurons is in line with the nature of the rest principle in that it amounts to a negative-feedback control increasing the input to neurons not getting enough, although the stimulation of growth goes beyond the actual definition of the principle. It seems likely that the second half of the principle (i.e., the weakening connections used too frequently) also may have an analogy in the withdrawal of neural processes when either they or their targets are used too much. This was briefly touched on in the previous section. Changeux and Danchin (1976) have pointed out that in development much of the final pattern of innervation in the nervous system seems to be accomplished by the removal of incorrect neurons and processes. At the time of neuroblast proliferation a large percentage (at least 75%, in tadpoles) of the neurons die out. Later, immediately after birth, there is a selective removal of about 60% of the neural projections to muscle end plates, (Brown, Jansen, & Van Essen, 1976) and about 40% of the climbing fiber connections onto Purkinjean cells in the cerebellum. As discussed earlier, however, there is some question as to whether the loss of functional synapses is due to withdrawal of the synaptic endings or to reductions in the amount of transmitter released.

The development and reduction of synapses appear to require a negative-feedback factor to suppress the synthesis of new receptors after innervation has occurred (Changeux & Danchin, 1976). Positive-feedback factors may also be required during development: This is suggested by the findings that presynaptic and postsynaptic toxins reduce the final number of functional connections. Toxins do not, however, block reinnervation in mature animals (Van Essen & Jansen, 1974), although synaptic remodeling and the apparent withdrawal of synapses still occur in adults (Brown & Ironton, 1976). This discrepancy between the results in developing and mature animals is in line with the hypothesis that a connection must be used first if rest is to cause an increase in strength. Administration of toxins before functional synapses are developed would prevent the lack of innervation and activity from stimulating the growth of connections, to the extent that the toxins are able to block the initial use of the synapses. In mature animals, the postsynaptic portions of the synapses have already been used before denervation and additional use would not be needed for rest to cause reinnervation.

In summary, the physiological evidence provides nearly unanimous support for the hypothesis that the strength of connections between neurons is regulated by negative rather than by positive feedback. Evidence for negative feedback has been found for every link in the chain of events occurring when one neuron influences the firing of a second (see Fig. 6.3).

The release of transmitter by the presynaptic neuron has been found to be under negative-feedback control for all systems studied, with the single exception of adrenergic synapses at very short time scales, and even this positive feedback is dominated by negative feedback at slightly longer time scales. Specific mechanisms for negative feedback, involving presynaptic receptors, are known for some systems, but more general factors, referred to as "fatigue," are also present. The reduction in the amount of transmitter released per action potential after persistent use can last for relatively long periods of time.

The amount of transmitter metabolized extraneuronally has been found to be reduced after denervation. This finding may, however, be artifactual, and it is unclear whether control at this link normally plays a role in the regulation of synaptic strength.

It has recently become clear according to Roth et al. (1977) that in "regulatory systems that use intracellular humoral signals [such] as neurotransmitters, immunoglobulins, cholesterol-containing serum lipoproteins" [and hormones, the] "target cells, rather than being passive recipients of humoral stimuli, are acting continuously to regulate their responsiveness to stimulation". High persistent concentrations of the humoral agents produce a decrease in the number of their receptors, whereas lack of the agents causes an increase in the number of their receptors. Only very few exceptions have been found to this negative-feedback rule, and, in systems using neuronal transmitter substances, the only known exception appears to be with serotonin, which relies instead upon receptor

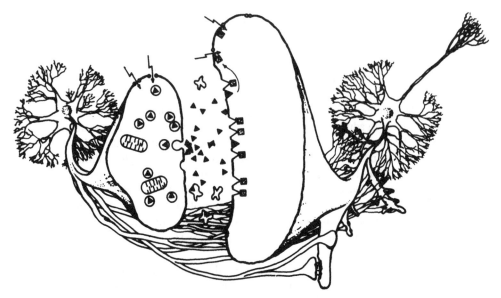

FIG. 6.3.   The connection between two neurons, with a close-up view of one synapse. The strength of the connection must be controlled by the following factors: (1) the amount of transmitter (black triangles) released by the presynaptic neuron on the left when an action potential (Z-shaped arrow) reaches a synapse; (2) the amount of transmitter removed in the synaptic cleft between the two neurons (e.g., by enzymes [the irregular four-lobed shapes in the cleft]); (3) the number of receptors (V-shaped indentations) on the postsynaptic neuron; (4) the affinity of these receptors (Notice the bottom receptor is too narrow for the transmitter); (5) the efficiency by which filling the receptors triggers electrical postsynaptic potentials (Z-shaped arrows) on the postsynaptic neuron, possibly through the actions of a second-messenger system (dotted squares); and (6) the total number of synapses (Notice the multitude of synapses in the background). None of these factors operates predominately in a positive-feedback manner as required by the use principle. Instead, there is strong evidence that most of them operate almost exclusively in a negative-feedback manner, in accordance with the rest principle.

affinity. Negative-feedback control of the number of receptors occurs with acetylcholine, norepinephrine, dopamine, prostaglandins, and GABA. The evidence is ambiguous at present for opiate receptors, and I know of no data yet for the remaining putative transmitters. Within the central nervous system it is clear that decreases in the amount of transmitter reaching the postsynaptic receptors cause an increase in the number of receptors, but the converse decrease after persistently high levels of transmitter has not yet been well established.

With the exception of the negative-feedback control with serotonin, there is as yet no evidence showing that changes in the receptor affinities have a role in regulating synaptic strength in neurons. In other cells responding to various neuronal transmitters, however, the affinity of the receptors does change, generally in a negative-feedback manner, so that persistent use reduces affinity, whereas disuse increases affinity. The only known exception is with acetylcholine receptors on nonneuronal targets that show positive cooperativity, responding preferentially to multiple inputs arriving within a short period of time. This positive feedback is also dominated by negative-feedback factors at longer time scales.

The available evidence suggests that the production of cyclic AMP hypothesized to act as a second-messenger system also is under negative-feedback control, showing greater responsiveness after disuse.

The roles played by the growth of neuronal processes, the production of new synapses, the loss of old synapses, and the withdrawal of processes remain rather speculative for adult animals. The growth and production of new synapses are clearly important during development and reinnervation. In these cases, the evidence suggests they work in a negative-feedback manner, increasing synapses to targets with little or no input. A positive-feedback factor may also be present, requiring that the synapses be used before they can be strengthened or maintained. It seems likely that withdrawal of synapses also occurs, but it cannot be stated with any confidence whether it works in a negative- or positive-feedback manner.

The two cases in which positive feedback has been clearly established both work on a very short time scale, and in both cases negative feedback predominates on a slightly longer time scale. This arrangement would be very useful because it would sharpen the information temporally in a manner akin to the sharpening produced spatially by lateral inhibition. By enhancing the response to multiple stimuli (i.e., to several inputs in a second), it can be shown that the system would incease its accuracy in filtering out noise coming from random inputs and in responding to real stimuli that produce multiple inputs.

This review has been restricted to an examination of findings at the synaptic level. Results obtained from systems containing several neurons, such as post-tetanic potentiation (Beswick & Conroy, 1965; Spencer & Wigdor, 1965), have not generally been covered. The reason for this is that systems of neurons do not necessarily reflect the rules governing synaptic plasticity. For instance, synapses become weaker with overuse, but a system with strong recurrent inhibition cannot be overused easily and will show little weakening. The system I call a *dopamine junction* actually becomes stronger with overuse. The possible roles of these and other systems are discussed at length in Chapters 9 and 10. The actions of these systems, however, seem to make sense only within the context of individual synapses obeying the rest principle.

I want to mention one final point about the physiological evidence that has implications for the rest principle. The experiments showing supersensitivity in neurons have involved both facilitory synapses using acetylcholine and inhibitory synapses using dopamine, norepinephrine, and GABA. This has implications for the definition of *rest* in the rest principle. For facilitory synapses, rest could mean the lack of any of the following: (1) filling of the receptors; (2) activation of second-messenger systems; (3) production of excitatory postsynaptic potentials; and (4) firing of the postsynaptic cell. For inhibitory synapses, rest could mean only the lack of: (1) filling of the receptors; (2) activation of second messenger systems, or (3) production of inhibitory postsynaptic potentials. Lack of firing by the postsynaptic neuron would not indicate rest for an inhibitory synapse. In the denervation and disuse studies with norepinephrine and GABA receptors, it is likely that the postsynaptic neurons fired more often than normal when they did not receive inhibitory input, and the result was an increase in the number of inhibitory transmitter receptors. This distinction between rest at the synaptic level and rest for the entire postsynaptic neuron must be kept in mind when trying to determine the consequences of the rest principle in systems where inhibitory connections are present.

The material covered in this chapter has been quite technical and, for many of you, may have been difficult to follow. To a large extent this was unavoidable. I wanted to cover all the physiological evidence relevant to the mechanisms controlling the strength of neural connections. Consequently, a wide range of diverse findings had to be examined. It was not possible to give a proper background here for an understanding of all these findings, nor was it possible to avoid technical terms.

Perhaps it would be helpful if the conclusions were stated in a somewhat different and hopefully more comprehensible way:

1. The strength of neural connections can be changed. Consequently, the changes in the strength of connections could form the basis for learning and memory storage.

2. The strength is changed as a function of use and disuse of the connections themselves. No external reinforcement mechanism is required.

3. There is no evidence for mechanisms that would increase the strength of connections the more they are used. There is no physiological support for the use principle.

4. Instead, nearly all the mechanisms make connections become weaker if the connections are overused and stronger if they are allowed to rest. In other words, the mechanisms act in a negative-feedback manner.

5. Pure negative-feedback control cannot explain behavioral results. It leads to absurd conclusions, such as that a response should become stronger the less often it is perfomed and weaker with each additional trial.

6. The rest principle is negative-feedback control with one addition: A connection must be used before it rests in order to become stronger; or, stated in another way, the rate of strengthening during the rest period is greatest shortly after use and reaches zero after very long periods of rest.

7. The rest principle is still in agreement with the physiological data and can account for behavioral results.

In Chapter 7 we return to examining how the rest principle explains behavioral findings. For most psychologists the area will be much more familiar than that covered in this chapter. We look at instrumental learning: How does reinforcement strengthen responses other than those already elicited by the reinforcing stimulus itself?

7 Instrumental Learning I: Drive and Stimulus Reduction

In previous chapters we have considered how neurons functioning according to the *rest principle* could account for various "mechanical" activities. Sharpening of contrast by lateral inhibition and organization of response changes are mechanical actions readily accomplished by electrical circuitry in television sets and servomechanisms. Classical conditioning is also easy to accept as a mechanical activity not requiring cognition: Peripheral reflexes can be conditioned even in humans with completely severed spinal columns (Ince, Bracker, & Alba, 1978).

We now begin covering topics, such as decision making, thinking, and feeling happy, for which neurophysiological explanations are inherently unacceptable to some people. The idea that neurons may be responsible for such actions even may provoke a strong negative emotional reaction. Perhaps the reason for this is a remnant of the homunculus (to use a neutral term) concept. As illustrated in Fig. 7.1, the modern homunculus probably has been, already, considerably crowded. Even the firm believers in "mind" have little trouble accepting neuronal processing of sensory input or response output. The position of the homunculus in the drawing is close enough to our own lives: listening to processed auditory input, watching processed visual input, and pushing buttons that elicit complex programmed actions, so that it is easy to agree that neurons could serve the homunculus as electronics serve us. Intuitively, the homunculus may still, however, be felt to be sitting in the midst, perceiving the sensory input, experiencing emotions, thinking, and making decisions. This chapter and Chapter 8 may not be able to do away with the homunculus, but at least they will crowd him a good deal more, by showing how many of these less mechanical functions would be accomplished by neurons employing the *rest principle*.

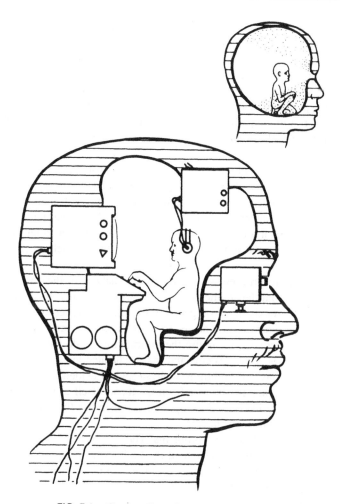

FIG. 7.1. The crowding of the modern homunculus.

A somewhat less supernatural approach admits that neurons are responsible for these functions but claims that the actions of the complex neuronal systems can be understood only by analyses at the system level and that a "molecular" analysis of the functioning of the individual neurons and synapses can contribute nothing to an understanding of complex behaviors. Psychology has not, however, become so sophisticated that is can prove that some postulate cannot be proved, as can be done, for instance, in mathematics. Therefore, the only honest way to determine the usefulness of a molecular analysis is to try it and see how well it can account for behavior.

One limitation of a molecular analysis is, however, already inherent in the previously presented conclusion about the rest principle: The effect of a particular input situation on the connections within a neuronal system is affected by how the neurons are arranged (i.e., by the cytological architecture). For example, strong continual stimulation of a simple pathway of facilitory neurons will, according to the principle, cause a great weakening of the connections. If, however, each neuron in the pathway has recurrent inhibition and turns itself off immediately after firing, the connections will be protected from any great loss of strength.

Our knowledge of the cytological architecture for most parts of the brain except the cerebellar cortex, the hippocampus, and some sensory systems is rather meager. This of course limits the accuracy of the present analysis. It is clear that there are major differences in the architecture of different parts of the brain. For instance, even at a gross level the mess found in the retucular system bears little resemblance to the orderly pattern found in the cerebellum (Eccles, 1967; Llinás, 1975).

There are two ways to proceed with a molecular analysis in the absence of complete information about the architecture of the various systems. First, we can ignore the effects of preexisting arrangements of different types of neurons, assuming only random innervation, and see to what extent one can nevertheless account for behavior. Second, we can use the information we do have about the cytological architecture of some systems and make educated guesses about that of other systems on the basis of preliminary physiological evidence, generalizations from other systems, and predictions from the theory itself as to the type of architecture that would be likely to develop. We can then use this "conceptual nervous system" to account for behavior.

Both of these approaches have their problems. The first starts with an assumption (uniform random innervation throughout the brain) known to be false. Empirical results are therefore bound to differ to some degree from the theoretical predictions. The second approach, on the other hand, has the limitation of allowing the theorist too much freedom. If one is allowed to assume a wide variety of hypothetical arrangements for the neurons in various parts of the brain and to stipulate arbitrarily which systems dominate in which situations, it should be possible to account for all existing behavioral data or, if desired, for all results opposite to the empirical data. The only way to determine the validity of the theory would then be to wait until physiological studies show whether the hypothetical cytological arrangements that account for the real behavioral data do in fact exist.

I use both of these approaches, although accepting their limitations. In this chapter and in Chapter 8, only random innervation is assumed, except for pathways such as $S_{h+\text{food}}-R_{\text{in}}$, which the theory has already predicted should develop strong lateral inhibitory output with daily experience. We then see how well the rest principle accounts for the general empirical findings concerning reinforcement and instrumental learning, acknowledging that a perfect match is impossible. In Chapter 9, I discuss how a few relatively reasonable assumptions regarding the cytological architecture of various systems can improve the precision of the match.

In the present chapter and Chapter 8 we examine the general category of instrumental learning. There are two distinguishing features of instrumental learning. First, unlike many other forms of learning, including most human verbal learning, there is a distinct reinforcing event such as the presentation of food or the termination of shock. Second, unlike classical conditioning, the response that is strengthened is not elicited by the reinforcing event itself. For instance, in classical conditioning with food as the reinforcer, the response measured is salivation, which is elicited by food. In instrumental learning, the response can be bar pressing, maze running, and so on—responses not automatically produced by the presentation of food. These distinctions are not perfect; both classical conditioning and learning without a distinct reinforcer have roles in many forms of instrumental learning. Nevertheless, the distinctions suffice for our purposes.

An artificial and inappropriate distinction between classical conditioning and instrumental learning, alluded to at the beginning of this chapter, is that instrumental learning is less mechanical and must be described in cognitive terms. This distinction appears to be primarily the result of our intuitive projections. For instance: Salivation seems to occur automatically; we do not decide to salivate. Consequently, we do not imagine the dog in a classical conditioning study to be engaged in decision-making or goal-directed behavior. In contrast, it is very easy to imagine the rat in a maze *deciding* which way to go, *being motivated* to run through the maze, and *having a goal* of reaching the food. Consequently, there is a tendency to assume that such mentalistic functions must be included in an explanation of instrumental learning.

The inadequacy of this distinction already has been clearly shown by various experiments, such as classical conditioning of what appear to be goal-directed behaviors and instrumental learning of autonomic responses. The most effective rebuff to this distinction, however, would be a demonstration that instrumental learning can be explained adequately without the introduction of any cognitive terms or mentalistic functions. This is possible with the rest principle. In physiological terms the explanation for instrumental learning is just as mechanical as that given in Chapter 4 for classical conditioning.

The rest principle can account for the basic phenomena in very simple ways that are also rather easy to comprehend. The analysis of each type of instrumental learning begins, therefore, with these simple explanations, which are also summarized in Table 7.1 for easy reference. In most cases, however, there are additional factors that would contribute to the behavior. Sometimes these merely give redundancy, thus providing additional mechanisms for assuring that a behavioral result already produced by the simple means will occur or will occur

TABLE 7.1.
Summary of How the Rest Principle Accounts for
Different Types of Instrumental Learning

1. *Positive reinforcement from drive reduction:* Drives are merely intense persistent internal stimuli, with well-learned consumatory responses that eliminate the drives while inhibiting extraneous sensory input and other responses. $S-R$ pathways that provide the appropriate stimuli for the consumatory response will be forced to rest while the consumatory response is being made and allowed to rest while the drive is satiated. Strengthening of the connections from the $S-R$ pathway to the neurons involved in producing the consumatory response also occurs, with limitations, by means of classical conditioning.

2. *Escape learning from intense stimuli:* Those $S-R$ pathways that eliminate their own intense S are allowed to rest after firing and therefore become stronger.

3. *Punishment of response with intense stimuli:* To the extent that the intense stimulus is able to increase reverberation in any portion of the $S-R$ pathway used just before or during its presentation, the pathway will be weakened. Classical conditioning of the preceding S to any well-established UCR elicited by the intense stimulus also may develop a competing response to the original R.

4. *Extinction of responses previously reinforced by drive reduction or escape from intense stimuli:* An $S-R$ pathway that had been strengthened by previous elimination of the S when R occurs will be used repeatedly when R no longer removes S and thus will be weakened.

5. *Active avoidance:* The connections between a signal, S_L, and a response, R, that prevents a strong stimulus, S_E, are strengthened in two ways: First, if the response terminates the signal and the strong stimulus during escape learning, the S_L-R, S_L-S_E, and S_E-R connections are all allowed to rest after use and become stronger. Subsequently, S_L alone may elicit R via S_L-R and S_L-S_E-R. Second, if R is already an UCR for S_E, the connections between S_L and the S_E-R pathway will be strengthened by classical conditioning. In addition, rebound general deactivation after S_E is escaped or avoided could contribute to the resting and growth of pathways just used.

6. *Positive reinforcement from intracranial stimulation:* The neurons producing intracranial self-stimulation are those representing the AND gate combination of an internal (drive) stimulus and the stimuli associated with removal of the drive (e.g., S_{h+food}). Pathways used just prior to the firing of these neurons will be strengthened during the inhibition-induced rest, as with drive reduction learning.

(continued)

more easily. In other cases they produce additional effects. Many of these mechanisms involve changes within the neuronal pathways that the rest principle predicts should occur with prolonged experience. The explanations for these mechanisms become somewhat complicated, but they do seem to give a closer approximation to reality.

Escape learning is discussed first because it is the simplest and most basic type of instrumental learning according to the rest principle. Imagine that a strong stimulus, such as electric shock is present and causing widespread activation of S_E neurons in the brain. These have random connections to various responses, including R_1, R_2, . . . , which do not stop the shock, and to R_{BP} (bar pressing), which does terminate shock. If the connections to R_1 happen to be strongest, S_E-R_1 will be emitted repeatedly until the connections are weaker than those of

TABLE 7.1.
(Continued)

---

7. *Positive reinforcement from stimulation of moderate intensity and duration:* There is an optimal level of firing for the strengthening of connections that has them fire, gain optimal advantage from the larger increments of strengthening occurring early in the rest period, then fire again, and so on. Consequently, there will be an optimal stimulus intensity for strengthening the connections in the involved pathways, the optimal point for intensity decreasing as the duration of stimulation increases. The $S-R$ pathways responsible for maintaining or producing optimal levels will be strengthened preferentially themselves and/or gain additional routes via $S-S$ and $R-S$ connections to the pathways firing optimally.

8. *Positive reinforcement from moderate changes in stimulus intensity:* Change itself can act as a stimulus, and thus there would be an optimal rate of change in stimulation for strengthening change-excited pathways. There also is an optimal duration of stimulation for increasing the strength of connections in the stimulation-excited pathways.

9. *Positive reinforcement from cognitive activities and motor activities:* No distinction is made between stimulus-input neurons and those involved in other activities: There is, therefore, an optimal rate of firing for the neurons involved in thinking and in producing motor responses.

10. *Positive reinforcement from moderate stimulus complexity, puzzle solving, and moderate rates of information flow.* Many neurons should arrange themselves into hierarchical pyramids, with the bottom neurons stimulated by common features of the input and feeding into higher neurons that are fired by progressively more complex and selective features. The top neurons are fired infrequently, so connections from them are strengthened whenever used. Stimuli with enough complexity to fire the top neurons, but not so much as to cause overuse of the bottom neurons, will cause a net increase in strength. There will be an optimal rate of stimulation presentation, which just allows each top neuron to be fired before the next stimulus is shown; because the time needed to reach the top neuron depends upon the complexity and novelty of each stimulus, there will be an optimal rate of information flow. Pyramids in which the bottom neurons are fired by cognitive input, such as solving mental puzzles and attempting to understand something, should function similarly. Strengthening will be increased by the development of routes through both the sensory and cognitive pyramids that allow the top neurons to be fired or of faster routes that minimize the firing of bottom neurons needed to fire the top ones.

S_E -R_2. Eventually the animal will work its way down through the various responses until it comes to R_{BP}. R_{BP} can be used only once because it terminates shock; therefore S_E -R_{BP} will rest after use and grow stronger.

This alone would assure that no other response could be stronger than R_{BP} after one escape trial: Any responses that initially had been stronger would have been weakened by repeated use. These responses, however, will still be approximately equal to R_{BP} in strength, because they would be reduced to about the level of R_{BP} only at the time that bar pressing terminated shock and allowed all connections to rest and grow. During the second trial, R_{BP} has a roughly equal chance of being anywhere in the sequence of those responses with the same strength. All responses that happen to be made before R_{BP} will gain in strength as much as R_{BP} does when shock is terminated, but the remaining responses that are not used again will show smaller increments because a long time has elapsed since they were last used. Thus the field of equal responses will be reduced progressively until R_{BP} happens to be used first and is the only response to receive the full increment in strength. Subsequently, the animal will continue to use R_{BP} to terminate shock as long as it is successful. Of course, if R_{BP} no longer stops S_E, S_E-R_{BP} will be used repeatedly until it is weaker than some other pathway (i.e., the response is extinquished).

The process of eliminating incorrect responses would be improved if either (1) there is any reverberation within those pathways partially maintained by S_E input or (2) there is overlap between the different S_E-R pathways, so that they share the same neurons.

Imagine that S_E-R_1, S_E-R_2, ... are complex pathways involving some reverberatory circuitry, so that neurons have the potential of indirectly adding to their own excitation (e.g., A–B–C–D–A). Lateral inhibitory connections have developed between the more frequently used input neurons to the complex portions and also between the output response neurons, so that only one pathway is maximally activated at a time and only one response emitted at a time. Within each pathway, once a critical level of excitation is reached, the reverberatory circuits will be able to continue firing by themselves for a short period of time. The presence of diffuse excitation from S_E will, however, allow the reverberation to continue much longer.

Such circuitry would tend to make first one pathway, S_E-R_1, be activated along with its reverberatory circuits; R_1 will continue to be emitted repeatedly. Eventually the input connections will be weaker than those to R_2, and then the reverberatory circuits of S_E-R_2 will be activated. Reverberation within S_E-R_1, however, will continue with the aid of diffuse excitation from S_E. The output from S_E-R_1 will probably be less than that of S_E-R_2, and the latter response will be made, but the continuing reverberation in S_E-R_1 will weaken the connections in it far below the level at which R_1 ceased to be the emitted response. Only the final successful pathway, S_E-R_{BP}, will be free of nearly all reverberation because it eliminates S_E and thus the diffuse excitation that maintained a high level of reverberation.

Within the series of responses the animal emits before reaching R_{BP}, reverberation would cause the first response to be weakened most, whereas the response immediately prior to R_{BP} would suffer little weakening because R_{BP} stops all reverberation shortly after this next-to-last response is made.

Now imagine that the pathways overlap so that some portions of S_E-R_1 are also in S_E-R_2, S_E-R_3, ... , S_E-R_{BP}. The amount of overlap can be shown to be roughly proportional to how close the responses are in order of emission. Reverberation in S_E-R_1 will contribute most to the firing of the pathway with which it shares the most overlap, so this is the response most likely to be used after S_E-R_1. Furthermore, once S_E-R_1 has been greatly weakened by reverberation, those pathways having the least overlap with it and thus containing fewest of its weakened units will be the most likely to be emitting responses. Use and reverberation of S_E–R_1 will thus tend in the long run to be most detrimental to the pathway whose response follows R_1 among the other pathways. Such overlap will cause more weakening to the middle responses in a series and least to the first and last responses, because a middle response (e.g., R_{10}) will have some parts weakened that overlap with the preceding responses (R_9, R_8, . . .) and other parts weakened by overlap with subsequent responses (R_{11}, R_{12}, . . .). The first response will suffer from overlap only with subsequent responses, and the last response will be weakened only by units shared with preceding responses.

Combining these two factors, we see that the response immediately preceding R_{BP} will have a net gain in strength almost, but not quite, as large as that for R_{BP}. Consequently, there is a fair chance that the animal may continue to emit it before R_{BP}, as is seen in "superstitious" learning. Pigeons, for example, who happen to turn around once before making the "correct" response of pecking a key and obtaining food, may continue to turn around before pecking. This also can help to account for the ability to learn a required series of responses.

Drive-reduction learning could be most simply treated as just another form of escape. Drives such as hunger and thirst are seen merely as internal stimuli that become intense during deprivation and cause widespread activation. Any response that terminates the stimulation will be allowed to rest after use and will become stronger, just as R_{BP} that terminated shock became stronger. Responses that do not remove the drive stimulation will be weakened by overuse just as in escape learning. This is, of course, what is described in Chapter 3 as an explanation for animals' learning to eat. Eating later was (Fig. 4.8) shown to be really a response chain: Learning of each component in the chain was partially reinforced by the eventual removal of hunger. Responses involved in food acquisition were included as part of this chain, and they too would be partially strengthened by removal of hunger.

In Fig. 4.8, you will notice that the response of searching for food stimuli was elicited by the stimulus $S_{h+\text{nonfood stimuli}}$. This is actually a rather peculiar stimulus: The "S_h" part is clear—it is simply input from hunger—but the "nonfood stimuli" part implies activation by the absence of stimuli related to food rather than by the presence of particular nonfood stimuli. In this way the $S_{h+\text{nonfood stimuli}}$ neurons, or $S_{h+\text{no food}}$ for short, are similar to the "off" neurons in the visual system activated by the absence of light stimulation. Nevertheless, this must be the stimulus for searching for food rather than merely S_h, otherwise the animal would continue searching for food-related stimuli after they already have been located and other responses such as approaching the food and eating it are needed. This is important to the present discussion because it shows another way, in addition to removal of hunger, by which food-acquisition response can be reinforced. Inasmuch as $S_{h+\text{no food}}$ is the stimulus for searching for food stimuli, the connections eliciting such responses also can be strengthened merely by the discovery of food stimuli. Once food stimuli are found, the stimulus $S_{h+\text{no food}}$

is removed, and the connections from this stimulus to the response that produced the food stimuli will be allowed to rest and grow stronger. The term *searching for food stimuli* is merely a general name for a very broad class of possible responses, including all those that might make food stimuli be perceived. For instance, in the laboratory, bar pressing that caused food to be given would fall in this class. $S_{h+no\ food} - R_{BP}$ would be strengthened first by the termination of $S_{h+no\ food}$ when food stimuli appeared and subsequently by the removal of S_h.

Reinforcement by drive reduction becomes somewhat more complicated in an older animal with well-developed consumatory responses. The removal of the drive stimulation and of the specific stimulus analogous to $S_{h+no\ food}$ still contributes to the learning, but other factors derived from the consumatory response also have a strong influence.

The response chain shown in Fig. 4.8 consisted primarily of pairs of opposing responses. Each pair had a common element in the stimuli eliciting the two responses and one stimulus element that was different for the responses. For instance, $R_{jaw\ lowered}$ and $R_{jaw\ raised}$ both were elicited partially by stimulation from hunger + food stimuli + food in mouth + dry and hard, but the former also required stimulation from the jaw's being up, whereas the latter required input from the jaw's being down. Clearly it would be beneficial to the animal if there were mutual inhibitory connections between the opposing responses and also between the stimuli eliciting them (e.g., it is easier to raise the jaw if the response of lowering it is strongly inhibited). In Chapter 5, I showed how lateral inhibitory connections develop automatically between parallel pathways with the rest principle; I now show why lateral inhibitory connections are particularly likely to be strengthened between such opposing responses because the inhibitory connections between $S_{h+no\ food}$ and S_{h+food} and between their responses are important for drive-reduction learning.

Imagine three stimuli, S_A, S_1, and S_B, that converge on two AND gates, S_{1A} and S_{1B}, which then elicit responses R_{1A} and R_{1B} (Fig. 7.2). Because both S_{1A} and S_{1B} receive input from S_1, and because R_{1A} removes S_A and produces S_B, it is almost certain that immediately after S_{1A} has fired, S_{1B} will fire and make S_{1A} rest through the lateral inhibitory connections. Similarly, S_{1A} almost always will be able to inhibit S_{1B}, R_{1A} will be able to inhibit R_{1B}, and R_{1B} will be able to inhibit R_{1A}. The only time this will not happen is when S_1 eventually disappears. Because the units in the opposing pathways nearly always rest after use, the inhibitory connections they excite will also be able to rest after firing and therefore will grow stronger according to the rest principle.

In contrast, imagine two pathways receiving input from completely independent stimuli. There is a good chance that the second pathway will not be active just after the first has been used once and therefore will not be able to inhibit the first or its inhibitory connections. Consequently, the lateral inhibitory connec-

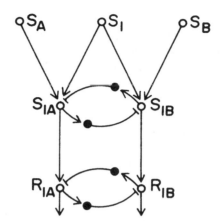

FIG. 7.2. Pathways that produce opposing responses and develop very strong mutual lateral inhibitory connections.

tions between independent pathways are much less likely to be strengthened than those between pathways producing opposing responses.

Now let us apply this to the neurons stimulated by hunger. S_1 is S_h, S_A represents food-related stimuli, S_B represents the absence of food stimuli, S_{1A} is $S_{h+\text{food}}$, S_{1B} is $S_{h+\text{no food}}$, R_{1A} is R_{in}, and R_{1B} is the class of responses that cause food stimuli to be perceived. We will be dealing with specific new responses in this class, such as R_{BP} (if bar pressing produces food), but it should be remembered that the experienced animal will already have general responses of this type being elicited by $S_{h+\text{no food}}$. Responses that increase the general sensory input, such as visual exploration and sniffing, will have allowed the animal in the past often to perceive existing food stimuli and thus are now elicited by $S_{h+\text{no food}}$. The internal response of sensory arousal will have had a similar effect and also will be produced. Moreover, there will be a general arousal of nonconsumatory motor responses, but the specific responses elicited by $S_{h+\text{no food}}$ will depend on the species and the individual animal's previous experience. Finally, the animal will possess strong inhibitory lateral connections between $S_{h+\text{no food}}$ and $S_{h+\text{food}}$ and between R_{in} and the general class of nonconsumatory motor and sensory arousal responses.

Let us now return to the rat's learning to bar press for food. The stimulus $S_{h+\text{no food}}$ elicits various responses. Incorrect responses (i.e., those that do not produce food-related stimuli) will be eliminated as before. When the rat finally presses the bar, the $S_{h+\text{no food}} - R_{BP}$ connections will be strengthened in several ways: (1) As before, presentation of food terminates $S_{h+\text{no food}}$ and allows the pathway to rest; (2) firing of $S_{h+\text{food}} - R_{\text{in}}$ actively inhibits $S_{h+\text{no food}}$ and all components of the $S_{h+\text{no food}} - R_{BP}$ pathway that previously have been involved often in producing food stimuli; (3) the responses increasing sensory input, including sensory arousal, will be inhibited, thus increasing the chances that the sensory components in the bar-pressing response will rest and their connections become stronger, (4) the general arousal of nonconsumatory responses will be inhibited, thus increasing the chances that the motor components in the R_{BP} response will rest; and finally (5) hunger will be removed when enough food has been eaten, so that $S_{h+\text{no food}} - R_{BP}$ will be allowed to rest for a long time.

In addition to having specific inhibitory connections to the $S_{h+\text{no food}}$ system, the $S_{h+\text{food}} - R_{\text{in}}$ pathway will have developed a strong inhibitory surround as a result of its frequent use in the past, as seen in Chapter 4. In that chapter, it is shown how this inhibitory surround, plus the removal of hunger, would strengthen facilitory connections from $S_{h+\text{bell}}$ onto the $S_{h+\text{food}} - R_{\text{in}}$ pathway itself during classical conditioning. By the same process, facilitory connections from $S_{h+\text{no food}} - R_{BP}$ to $S_{h+\text{food}} - R_{\text{in}}$ would be strengthened. Of course, inhibitory connections would also be growing between the two pathways as they did in the example shown in Fig. 7.2, and the inhibitory connections generally would be stronger than the facilitory. A similar phenomenon was found in a simulation of lateral inhibition: Facilitory connections would grow between parallel pathways as long as the inhibitory connection predominated. Facilitory connections could contribute to a rebound firing of $S_{h+\text{food}} - R_{\text{in}}$ after $S_{h+\text{no food}} - R_{BP}$ was used, particularly if their input took longer to reach $S_{h+\text{food}} - R_{\text{in}}$, for instance, as a result of its coming via a multisynaptic route. The general result will be a close coupling of the two pathways, so that one or the other will be able to dominate nearly all pathways not related to eating whenever hunger is sufficiently strong, and so that when one ceases to fire, the other is very likely to fire even in the absence of the appropriate input. For instance, any pause in the firing of $S_{h+\text{no food}} - R_{BP}$ will elicit some rebound firing of $S_{h+\text{food}} - R_{\text{in}}$, even when food is not present. Furthermore, to use anthropomorphic terms, if the rat happens to "think" about bar pressing, its next thought is almost certainly going to be of obtaining food and eating. Conversely, thoughts of food would elicit thoughts of bar pressing. Priming an animal with a small amount of food would therefore help to start a mildly hungry animal bar pressing. While it is responding, expectations of food would help to direct its behavior.

So far we have neglected the stimuli other than hunger that are present when an animal is learning an instrumental response. In order to symbolize such stimuli, imagine that there is a signal lamp (L) stimulating S_L units in the brain and also helping to stimulate $S_{L+h+\text{no food}}$ units when the animal is hungry and no food is available. Any connections from these units to R_{BP} will also be strengthened when food is presented. $S_{L+h+\text{no food}} - R_{BP}$ will be allowed to rest by removal of $S_{h+\text{no food}}$, by inhibition from $S_{h+\text{food}} - R_{\text{in}}$, by removal of general sensory and motor arousal, and by the eventual termination of hunger. $S_L - R_{BP}$ will be strengthened by the removal of arousal and inhibition of its components near R_{BP}, but it is limited in strength; once it has become strong enough to elicit bar pressing by itself when the animal is satiated, it can be used repeatedly without being interrupted by eating and thus will be weakened again.

The $S_{L+h+no\ food}$ $-R_{BP}$ pathway becomes very important if the experimenter causes the bar to produce food only when the signal lamp is lit. All other pathways to R_{BP} can be used repeatedly without being stopped by eating and thus will be weakened, but $S_{L+h+no\ food}$ $-R_{BP}$ always will rest after use and will be strengthened to the point where the rat is very likely to press the bar only when the light is on, it is hungry, and there is no food available. This pathway also will become coupled to S_{h+food} $-R_{in}$ and will be able to elicit expectations of food and eating. Such expectations may be important for increasing the internal intensity of the signal lamp so that the responses connected with it will be able to dominate other responses unrelated to eating.

Before we leave drive-reduction learning, it should be mentioned that there remains a class of factors contributing to this learning that has not yet been considered. As discussed further in chapter 8, providing pathways with rest is not the only requirement for making them become stronger; they also must be used before resting. In the present chapter we are considering pathways with high rates of activity so reinforcement occurs when rest is provided. There clearly are many pathways, however, that are used infrequently; rest comes automatically for them, and the use requirement is critical for their growth. In the food reward example here, such pathways would include those stimulated by the specific taste, smell, and appearance of the food. Less obviously, there are also neurons excited by complex features of the learning situation and by the solution of the mental puzzle, "How can I find food?", that the rat faces. Providing excitation to such infrequently used pathways and neurons will also help to reinforce bar pressing. Further discussion of these factors can be done properly, however, only after the bases for stimulus acquisition learning have been presented.

As an introduction to active-avoidance learning, let us return for a moment to escape learning. As occurred with drive reduction, other stimuli such as S_L can also play a role in escape learning. For instance, if bar pressing terminated shock, S_E, only when S_L were present, S_{L+E} $-R_{BP}$ would be strengthened. If R_{BP} also terminated S_L, the S_L $-R_{BP}$ pathway also would be strengthened to the point where S_L alone would cause the animal to bar press. If bar pressing only terminated S_L and the rat never received shock, the animal might learn to bar press, but it might learn more easily, for instance, merely to turn away from the light. When R_{BP} terminates both S_E and S_L, however, the rat is almost certain to use R_{BP}, because turning away from the light does not remove shock, and S_L $-R_{BP}$ could become quite strong.

Having S_L $-R_{BP}$ strong enough to elicit bar pressing by itself might be seen as explaining active-avoidance learning, in which an animal makes a response when a signal is given, thus preventing presentation of an aversive strong stimulus. Preliminary training generally is done with escape learning, in which the aversive stimulus is preceded by the onset of the signal. The animal first learns to make the response in order to escape the aversive stimulus, then begins to make it to the signal alone, and thus avoids the aversive stimulus.

There are, however, several problems with this idea: (1) S_L alone is only a weak stimulus and by itself is unlikely to be able to determine the animal's behavior; the animal might be more likely to use S_{itch}–R_{scratch} rather than S_L–R_{BP} regardless of how strong the connections are from S_L to R_{BP}, because S_{itch} dominates S_L. (2) Animals can, although usually with difficulty, learn avoidance responses that do not terminate the signal stimulus. (3) The diffuse excitation from S_E could weaken any parts of the S_L–R_{BP} pathway it caused to be overused during the period that S_E is present. These problems are confirmed by the empirical evidence. It is extremely difficult to train rats to bar press in order to avoid shock; even after hundreds of trials they are able to avoid only a small percentage of the shocks (Biederman, D'Amato, & Keller, 1964).

As Bolles (1970, 1971) and Mackintosh (1974, pp. 303, 340–342) point out, active avoidance is learned easily only when the required response is automatically elicited by the strong aversive stimulus. Running and leg withdrawal, for instance, are UCRs for general and specific shock UCSs respectively and therefore are readily learned as avoidance responses.

These responses are likely to have been used successfully by the animal many times in the past for terminating painful tactual stimulation, and although genetic factors cannot be eliminated, this could account for their being elicited by shock. In any case, the pathways producing these responses are well-established and would have developed strong inhibitory surrounds. Consequently, a pathway such as S_E–R_{run} will be able to cause classical conditioning of preceding stimuli. For instance, the connections from S_L to S_E, to R_{run}, and to intermediate neurons in the S_E–R_{run} pathway will be strengthened if S_L precedes S_E, just as the $S_{h+\text{bell}}$–$(S_{h+\text{food}}$–$R_{\text{in}})$ connections were strengthened in Chapter 4. The growth of S_L–$(S_E$–$R_{\text{run}})$ does not depend entirely upon running being able to terminate shock, but if running does not stop it, the ability of S_L to elicit R_{run} will be weakened to the extent that S_E–R_{run} is weakened and the animal produces other responses to S_E. Furthermore, just as some of the strengthening of $S_{h+\text{bell}}$–$(S_{h+\text{food}}$–$R_{\text{in}})$ occurred because eating eventually terminated S_h, some of the strengthening of S_L–$(S_E$–$R_{\text{run}})$ will occur because running terminated shock and allowed the pathways to rest.

In addition to allowing S_L to elicit R_{run}, classical conditioning will also strengthen the connections from S_L to S_E. Whether the resulting excitation of central S_E units without the firing of tactual input neurons amounts to "conditioned fear" or whether it is necessary to invoke an internal UCR of fear, remains to be seen. Nevertheless, S_L will no longer be a weak stimulus able to stimulate mildly only a small number of neurons; it now will cause widespread excitation through the S_E units. Consequently, S_L will have no problem dominating, for instance, S_{itch}, and will be able to control behavior reliably.

Once S_L is established as a strong stimulus internally, a second component of active-avoidance learning becomes important. As we have seen before with escape learning, any response that terminates an intense stimulus will be strengthened. If the avoidance response (e.g., R_{run}) terminates S_L, the $S_L - R_{run}$ connections will be able to rest after use and will therefore be further strengthened. This would be particularly useful for shaping the response beyond the UCR elicited by shock. For instance, S_E causes running but does not specify where the rat is to run. If the required response is, for instance, running from one part of a shuttle box to the other, classical conditioning would cause S_L to elicit running in general, but termination of S_L when the rat reached the safe side of the shuttle box would be largely responsible for strengthening the responses directing the rat into the safe part of the shuttle box. Consequently, having the response terminate the signal greatly improves avoidance learning in such a situation (Kamin, 1957; Mowrer & Lamoreaux, 1942), but has little effect when the required response is running in an activity wheel (Bolles, Stokes, & Younger, 1966). In the latter situation the avoidance response is simply the UCR and there is no need to specify where to run.

In anticipation of Chapter 9, it might be mentioned that the establishment of S_L as an intense internal stimulus also would occur in the absence of classical conditioning if one portion of the brain were immune to weakening of connections with overuse. If the cerebral cortex, for instance, were very well supplied with recurrent inhibition by which neurons suppressed their own firing after each activation, the connections between neurons representing S_L and S_E would be strengthened merely by having been presented in close temporal proximity. Subsequently, S_L would excite the S_E units in the cortex and these would activate the S_E units in more plastic areas of the brain without strong recurrent inhibition. Any response that then terminated S_L would be strengthened, regardless of whether it were already an UCR for S_E. Consequently, the more important the cerebral cortex was in influencing the behavior of an animal, the easier it would be for responses that were not UCRs to the aversive stimulus to be learned as avoidance responses. Human subjects, for instance, have no difficulty learning to bar press in order to avoid shock (Turner & Solomon, 1962). The difference between people and rats may be related to the fact that for a quadruped, bar pressing is in opposition to the UCR of running; this is less so for a biped: Even human subjects are unable to learn an avoidance response that is in direct opposition to a well-established UCR (Turner & Solomon, 1962). Nevertheless, the large role that avoidance responses play in our everyday lives (e.g., stopping at red lights, putting on a coat before going outside) and the ease with which new avoidance responses are learned suggest that some structural difference between our brains and those of rats may be involved.

Even without resorting to cortical representation, the rest principle predicts that it would be possible for rats to learn to bar press to avoid shock, although it would take much longer than learning responses that are already UCRs. The only distinction between R_{BP} and R_{run} was assumed to be that $S_E - R_{run}$ was well-established and developed a strong inhibitory surround. If a rat were given sufficient escape training with bar pressing for $S_E - R_{BP}$ to become well-established and develop an inhibitory surround, $S_E - R_{BP}$ could also strengthen connections from S_L onto itself by classical conditioning and thus produce avoidance bar pressing.

With drive-reduction learning it was mentioned that part of the reinforcement was produced by the general inhibition of activity in sensory and motor pathways not involved in the consumatory response. This can be seen in reduced evoked potentials to stimuli, the suppression of the orienting response, or, out of the laboratory, in the difficulty of distracting a hungry animal when it is eating, and the very low probability that any other response will interrupt eating in the early stages. Shock and other painful or intense stimuli produce a diffuse excitation, as stated previously, that can be seen in EEG records and is also reflected in a general increase of blood flow in the brain (Lassen, Ingvar, & Skinkøj, 1978; Maximilian, Risberg, & Prohovniki, 1977). If, as a rebound, there is a general reduction of neural activity after escape or avoidance of shock, this also would contribute to the strengthening of the pathways producing the escape or avoidance response, as it does in drive-reduction learning.

The extreme resistance of avoidance learning to extinction that usually has been found has attracted considerable theoretical attention. The classic example involved dogs trained in a shuttle box to avoid shock: The animals showed no signs of the response weakening even after 200 trials without shock (Solomon, Kamin, & Wynne, 1953). Although other studies have shown extinction of avoidance responses, it nevertheless can be concluded that the resistance to extinction is very high.

In the usual paradigm in which the response terminates the signal stimulus, such resistance would be expected in the present analysis because the response is still terminating an internally intense stimulus, which is in itself reinforcing. Provided that the signal maintains its ability to elicit S_E activity, there should be even an improvement in performance, as actually seen in the study by Solomon et al. Even if the animal is trained in an avoidance situation in which the response does not terminate the physical presence of the signal, it is quite possible that the occurrence of the response changes the internal representation of the stimulus along the lines suggested by Soltysik (1963). If the animal dissociated the ''signal before the response'' from ''signal after the response,'' only the former is ever followed with shock and only it will have its connections to S_E strengthened. Of course, the response, by definition, terminates the former ''signal before the response.'' So even in this situation the behavior should be resistant to extinction.

Relatively rapid loss of the avoidance response can be produced, however, in various ways. If the animal is prevented from making the response, for instance, with curare or by locking the door of the shuttle box during extinction, the $S_L - S_E$ connections will be fired repeatedly and thus weakened. The removal of the ability of S_L to activate S_E will return S_L to being only a weak stimulus without the power to control the animal's behavior reliably (e.g., S_{itch} might again be able to dominate it). Thus the avoidance response will become much less probable, as has been found (Mackintosh, 1974, p. 336). Similarly, for animals trained with the response terminating the signal and thus not learning to dissociate the signal before and after the response, having the signal continue after the response during extinction training will cause overuse and weakening of the S_L-S_E connections. Consequently, the probability that the response will be made is reduced as a function of how long S_L continues after the response has been made, again in agreement with empirical findings (Katsev, 1967).

In the absence of such manipulations, an avoidance response can still be extinguished slowly despite the strengthening caused by the termination of the signal. This again involves the S_L-S_E connections. It will be remembered that these originally were strengthened partially by the inhibitory surround of the S_E-R_{run} pathway. In order for a conditioned response requiring more than momentary activation of the response-initiating neurons to be emitted, the CS must not activate the UCS–UCR pathway so strongly that it produces enough firing of the inhibitory surround to prevent its own influence on the pathway. Consequently, connections established by classical conditioning are not self-strengthening and in the absence of the UCS will be extinguished, as seen in Chapter 4. The S_L-S_E connections may receive some help from the termination of S_L when the response is made and by any rebound reduction in arousal. The latter, however, is probably rather weak when S_E is only partially activated (as opposed to full activation by the presentation of shock), and the diffuse excitation of S_E units probably results in some reverberation and weakening despite the removal of S_L. Another factor contributing to the weakening of S_E-S_L connections is the inherent variability in the latency for producing the avoidance response. Competing stimuli and responses may occasionally delay the avoidance response. During the longer interval, the S_L-S_E connections that are activated will be fired repeatedly and suffer rather much weakening. This starts a chain reaction, because the weakening produced by the occasional delay in responding will make S_L a less intense stimulus internally and render it more vulnerable to domination by other stimuli. This domination will cause more and longer delays, which then weaken the internal intensity of S_L further. Eventually, S_L is reduced to being only a weak stimulus and consequently, as stated before, the probability that the avoidance response will be made is decreased.

It is very easy to remove avoidance responses by shocking the animal when it does make the response rather than when it fails to make the response. This brings us to another topic: the use of punishment.

When a strong stimulus, such as S_E, is applied during or after a response, there are several ways in which the response could be weakened. There are also, however, requirements that must be met before each of these processes would be effective. If these requirements are not considered, punishment will be comparatively unreliable.

At the simplest level, a strong stimulus can stop an ongoing response merely by changing the stimulus situation. Imagine an animal in a nonaroused state casually exploring a maze. When shock is applied, a large number of neurons that were not previously active now are excited, eliciting responses such as jumping or running. The shock-elicited responses themselves may suppress incompatible responses, whereas the diffuse excitation may interfere with the coordination and sequential firing needed to make some responses. (Consider, for instance, the sequential requirements for production of the R_{in} response chain shown in Fig. 4.8.) To the extent that the neurons firing after the termination of shock are still different from those active before shock, first by continuing arousal and then perhaps by rebound reduction in arousal, the previously emitted responses will not reappear. This change in the stimulus situation by itself produces only a short-term suppression of preceding responses and does not explain the long-term weakening also usually seen.

The long-term weakening may be explained in two ways. The first is that the diffuse excitation from the strong stimulus causes overuse and weakening of some of the connections involved in the production of the preceding response. The running seen during shock, for instance, may be partially a reflection of overactivation of the pathways previously involved in casual walking. Overuse seems more likely, however, on the stimulus side, because the stimuli present just prior to shock, such as the sight of that part of the maze, are still present during shock. During the casual exploration of the maze when the animal was at the intersection preceding the place where shock was given, it received stimuli from both arms of the maze but those attracting it to the shock area must have been stronger, as evidenced by the fact that the animal went in that direction. On the trial after shock was given, the attractive input from the shock arm will have been weakened by the overuse of these stimulus units during application of S_E. Consequently the attractive input from the alternative arm will dominate, and the animal will enter it instead of the arm where shock was given. (How stimuli can be "attractive" is discussed in Chapter 8.) It should be pointed out here, however, that the weakening that reduces attraction is not contradictory to the increased internal intensity of the stimulus due to classical conditioning to S_E, discussed later: The former involves weakening of connections to infrequently used complex neurons, whereas the latter involves increased excitation of frequently used neurons.

It has been argued that because performance spontaneously improves after the termination of punishment trials, the suppression of responding caused by punishment could not have been due to a weakening of connections (e.g., Estes, 1944). As seen in Chapter 4, however, partial spontaneous recovery is inherent in the rest principle and occurs whenever connections that have been weakened by overuse are allowed to rest. The reason for this distinction between Estes' view and the rest principle is that Estes was obviously considering a static system in which neuronal connections are passive recipients of strengthening or weakening from external causes, whereas in the rest principle the changes are caused by a dynamic process within the connections. In a static passive theory, if punishment reduced the strength of connection X below that of Y, X would be otherwise identical to Y and would remain weaker unless some other external factor caused it to get stronger. In the dynamic process of the rest principle, if punishment caused X to be weakened by overuse whereas Y had not been used for a very long time and maintained a strength greater than X, there are two differences between X and Y: (1) At the present moment X is weaker than Y; and (2) X has just been tired, which is the prerequiste for subsequent strengthening; therefore, if both were then allowed to rest, X would show larger increments in strength than Y and eventually might well become stronger than Y.

In order for this first process to weaken a response, it is of course necessary that connections eliciting the response are activated by the strong stimulus more than those involved in competing responses. This might be likely to occur if the response is still being made when shock is applied, if the stimuli generally are still the same (except for the addition of S_E) or if reverberation is still present within the pathway producing the response. In all of these situations there is more activity in the S–R pathway of the punished response than in other pathways. If S_E added equally to the activity of all pathways, the result would be more detrimental to the pathway that already was excited. Furthermore, the diffuse excitation from S_E might be subthreshold for many units in nonactive pathways but above threshold in the pathway of the preceding response because of the added input from existing activity. The selective overuse of connections in the pathway of the preceding response would cause it to be weakened relative to other competing response pathways.

Punishment applied relatively long after the response and in a different stimulus situation would not be able to weaken the response selectively. Furthermore, there is a possibility that a strong stimulus, although inherently aversive, actually might strengthen the preceding response by altering the stimulus situation and thus removing excitation to the pathway producing the response. Objectively, the stimulus could be judged to be aversive because a response elicited by the stimulus that terminated it would be strengthened, but responses that did not terminate the stimulus would be weakened. Nevertheless, the stimulus might be specific enough so that it did not overlap the units eliciting the previously occurring response and would be ineffective as punishment. To the extent that the units activated by the strong stimulus and the responses connected with it suppress input from other stimuli or inhibit firing in other neurons, the pathway producing the preceding response would be strengthened. The relative amount of diffuse, as opposed to specific, excitation produced by a strong stimulus depends on the cytological architecture of the neuronal network involved, as well as the changes within the network previously caused by experience. Consequently, the present analysis, which is based upon the assumption of initially random connections, is inherently limited in its ability to specify which aversive stimuli would effectively weaken preceding responses by this process. It does seem likely, however, that as the physical intensity of the stimulus is increased beyond the point at which the specific excitation is saturated, the relative amount of diffuse excitation would be raised for nearly any network. Consequently, the not very surprising prediction, that the effectiveness of punishment is directly related to stimulus intensity (see Azrin & Holz, 1966), could be made; this prediction also, of course, could be made on several other grounds. It also seems likely that strong stimuli that have been frequently encountered in the past and for which the animal has well-established escape responses should be less effective for weakening preceding responses by this first process, but this is countered by the fact that such stimuli will be more effective by the second process.

This second process by which punishment could produce long-term weakening of a response is closely related to active avoidance. Consider the situation in which a rat has learned to bar press for some reward (e.g., food) and then the bar is electrified. Initially, as a result of the drive-reduction training, visual stimuli from the bar, S_{VB}, elicit approach and extension of the paw to the bar; then the tactual stimuli, S_{TB}, help elicit pressing. The animal now touches the bar and receives shock to the paw, which automatically elicits withdrawal of the paw, R_W. As in active avoidance learning classical conditioning strengthens S_{VB}-$(S_E$-$R_W)$ and S_{TB}-$(S_E$-$R_W)$. Withdrawing the paw is of course in opposition to the extending needed as a component of R_{RP}. Thus, bar pressing will be prevented by elicitation of R_W by S_{VB}. Furthermore, S_{VB} and S_{TB} and all other stimuli related to bar are now connected to S_E and represent strong internal stimuli, so any response that terminates them will be strengthened. R_W terminates S_{TB}, so S_{TB}-R_W would become stronger for this reason as well as by classical conditioning, if the animal advanced so far as touching the bar again. Turning away from the bar terminates S_{VB}, so this response might also become stronger; whether this happens, however, will depend on the extent of previous drive reduction training, the current intensity of hunger, and the possibility of other responses, such as escaping from the Skinner box, which would also terminate S_{VB} and other stimuli now connected to S_E. During the training for food, moving away from the bar was weakened as a response to S_h because it did not terminate hunger; the opposing response of approaching the bar became connected to the S_h units, and the ability of approach to dominate turning away would also have been strengthened. The presence of hunger after shock has been applied may prevent the animal from moving away from the bar in order to terminate the stimulation. Only a new response, not weakened during appetitive training and not directly opposed to approach (e.g., escaping from the Skinner box) is likely to be made. Hunger also will have developed strong connections to stimuli in the reinforcement situation. Its presence when shock is applied may be sufficient to make all parts of the Skinner box become associated with shock, and its subsequent presence will help elicit those stimuli that evoke S_E, thus further increasing the chances that the animal will "escape from the field."

This second process weakens a response essentially by active-avoidance reinforcement of competing responses. Consequently, it would predict that punishment of a response elicited by shock itself would not only be ineffective but would actually increase the strength of the response. This has in fact been found in some studies (Brown, 1969; Fowler & Miller, 1963; Morse, Mead, & Kelleher, 1967; Walters & Glazer, 1971). On the other hand, this situation would be very conducive to weakening of responses by the first process, because the same pathways used to elicit the initial response are being overused when punishment is present. Consequently, if the duration of the punishment stimulus is long enough or the intensity high enough (to assure a large amount of reverberation), so that the first factor could assure enough weakening by overuse to overcome the effects of the second factor, punishment should again be found to suppress the response. The empirical evidence shows that this is just what happens (Azrin, 1970; Misanin, Campbell, & Smith, 1966). In the two most comparable studies, Melvin and Anson (1969) punished aggressive displays in Siamese fighting fish with mild shock and found an increase in the response, whereas Fantino, Weigele, and Lancy (1972) punished the aggressive display with more intense shock and found a suppression of the response, preceded by a small increase.

The processes are partially complementary, the first being most effective in situations in which the second fails and vice versa. As seen in the foregoing, punishment of responses elicited by shock is not effective by the second process but the response can be weakened by the first process if the intensity is high enough. The second process is most effective for aversive stimuli with well-developed UCRs that are not very effective with the first process. The first process should predominate in organisms with very little experience with similar aversive stimuli, whereas the second should predominate in those with a large amount of such experience.

There are, however, gaps in the coverage by the two processes: situations in which neither is effective and punishment does not work. One example was just mentioned: punishment of shock-elicited responses with only moderate intensities of shock. A related example is the failure of spanking a dog to weaken its tendency to run away, if the spanking is applied without too much force as the dog is trying to run away (as my neighbors would testify). Another gap is illustrated by the fact that a response elicited primarily by one sensory modality should be difficult to punish with a relatively strong stimulus in another modality that has no well-developed UCRs. For instance, a terribly bad, but novel, smell presented only during the interval between courses at an elaborate dinner may suppress eating of the next course; the same smell presented only during intermission at a concert would be much less likely to keep people from listening to and enjoying the music after intermission. Finally, neither punishment process is generally effective if a relatively long time has elapsed and the stimulus situation has changed before the aversive stimulus is applied. The only way in which such postponed punishment could weaken a response is if some of the connections involved in producing the response were reactivated when punishment was delivered. This can, however, occur. It seems likely that special systems have evolved for doing this for pathways connecting food-related stimuli to eating, so that long-latency nausea can suppress the future intake of specific foods (i.e., conditioned taste aversions). In humans, verbal descriptions of the offense immediately prior to or during the delivery of punishment also might be able to suppress the misbehavior in the future. There even might be some truth in the adage "Let the punishment fit the crime," because the similarity could reactivate some of the connections originally involved in producing the crime.

Superficially it might seem more appropriate to cover the topic of working for intracranial stimulation, ICSS, in Chapter 8, which deals with reinforcement from increasing stimulation. Although factors discussed in Chapter 8 may play a minor role in ICSS, on closer examination ICSS is seen to be quite closely related to drive-reduction learning.

Stimulation of the brain areas in which ICSS is most effective often produces consumatory behaviors, such as eating or drinking. Conversely, lesions of these sites may produce adipsia and aphagia (failure to drink and eat). On the other hand, animals will work to escape electrical stimulation of brain areas, such as the ventromedial hypothalamic nucleus, in which stimulation suppresses eating by hungry animals. Lesioning of this area causes overeating and the development of gross obesity.

These findings, although relating ICSS to drives, also seemed to create a paradox. It looked as if the animals would work to increase hunger or thirst and to escape satiety. A generation of psychologists had been indoctrinated with the idea that drive reduction, not drive production, was positively reinforcing. Perhaps for this reason, many researchers tried (in vain) to find evidence that it was the termination of the electrical stimulation to the positive ICSS areas that was rewarding.

The solution to this paradox, as detailed by Rolls (1975) is that the rewarding brain areas for ICSS contain AND gate neurons, such as S_{h+food}, which are fired by the combination of the drive state (e.g., hunger) plus the stimuli signalling the item (e.g., food) that can remove the drive. For instance, firing in rewarding lateral hypothalamic areas can be elicited naturally by hunger plus the smell, sight, or taste of food or even by the sight of the syringe from which the monkeys had received glucose. As we have seen before, these AND gate neurons are responsible for triggering the consumatory responses: The simulations in Chapter 3, for instance, show how the $S_{h+food}-R_{in}$ pathway grows preferentially with experience according to the rest principle. Consequently, if the experimenter electrically or chemically stimulates S_{h+food}, the animal will eat if possible, even if it has just finished a large meal. Conversely, lesioning S_{h+food} units removes the trigger for R_{in}, and the animal is aphagic.

Despite the intuitive appeal and Rolls' evidence that the combination of, for example, hunger plus food is rewarding, it has not been previously shown elsewhere how the firing of S_{h+food} units strengthens the pathway producing the preceding response. According to the rest principle this occurs primarily because the inhibitory output from $S_{h+\text{food}}$ suppresses firing in other neurons. The details of the process are, of course, discussed at the beginning of this chapter, because it is the firing of $S_{h+\text{food}}$ units that was the major cause of drive-reduction learning with food reward. The only difference is that there is a second factor, the removal of hunger, that helps make the previously used pathway rest and become stronger.

With drive-reduction learning, rest for the previous response pathway is assured because firing of $S_{h+\text{food}}$ removes activation of sensory and motor pathways not involved in the consumatory act. During ICSS it has also been found that evoked potentials in sensory areas are suppressed (Ball, 1967). Evidence that nonconsumatory motor activity is also suppressed is more difficult to ascertain, because the appropriate stimuli for completion of the consumatory response chain are not present. If $S_{h+\text{food}}$ units are stimulated and there is no food *nearby* to eat, the response elicited (Fig. 4.8) is going to the food stimuli; in the absence of localized food stimuli this appears as stimulus-bound locomotor activity. This does not, however, mean that locomotor activity (e.g., maze running) could not be used as the required response for ICSS if we assume that the program for running is separate from the areas involved in deciding what response to make and that the running program can be triggered by different competing outputs from the decision areas. This seems quite reasonable: For instance, locomotor activity occurs when hungry rats (with no food stimuli present) search for food stimuli, when hungry rats approach food, and when rats that are not hungry engage in various activities. Consequently R_{walk} can be triggered by S_h, by $S_{h+\text{food}}$, and by other inputs not related to food, which I will call S_{other}. Before electrical stimulation, $S_{\text{other}}-R_{\text{walk}}$ is firing; during the electrical stimulation $S_{h+\text{food}+\text{no food near}}-R_{\text{walk}}$ is firing and $S_{\text{other}}-R_{\text{walk}}$ is resting, as evidenced by the suppression of evoked potentials, even though the response program itself is not inhibited but rather activated. Because of the rest, $S_{\text{other}}-R_{\text{walk}}$ is strengthened and the probability is increased that the rat will resume walking after brain stimulation, in response to S_{other}. The response program itself is probably protected from much weakening despite the continual use by redundant pathways and recurrent lateral inhibition, as discussed in Chapter 9.

Support for this conclusion that the pathways strengthened when walking through a maze produces brain stimulation are different from the pathways producing the locomotor activity during the electrical stimulation comes from experiments comparing the roles of dopamine (DA) and norepinephrine (NE). Stimulus-bound locomotion elicited by electrical stimulation of the lateral hypothalamus is believed to be mediated largely by NE pathways (Ettenberg & Milner, 1977; Rolls, 1975, pp. 79-86). When maze running is used as the required response for lateral hypothalamic ICSS, the behavior is dependent on DA pathways and not NE pathways (White, Brown, & Yachnin, 1978). Blocking of the DA pathways suppressed maze running for ICSS. Blocking of the NE pathways actually produced a small amount of increase in the maze running for

ICSS, thus suggesting that the NE pathways and their stimulus-bound locomotor activity subtracted normally from running for brain stimulation, as would be expected because of the continual activation of the R_{walk} response program. In contrast, when tail movements were the required response for lateral hypothalamic stimulation, the behavior was more dependent on the NE pathways, and blocking them greatly reduced ICSS. This also shows that there is no one transmitter substance responsible for all reinforcement. Both NE and DA are inhibitory (but in a peculiar way, as discussed in Chapter 10) and could easily help to make pathways rest and become stronger, but so could GABA and other inhibitory transmitters according to the rest principle. Furthermore, reinforcement also could be produced by a reduction in the release of facilitory transmitters. Evidence that transmitters other than DA and NE are also involved in ICSS can be seen also in the results obtained by White et al. (1978) and from many other studies, because the blocking of both DA and NE pathways did not abolish ICSS.

One peculiarity of intracranial self-stimulation is that animals will learn to make one response to turn on the electrical stimulation and another to terminate it (Hodos, 1965; Roberts, 1958). This initially was thought to indicate that the stimulation became aversive with longer durations. Although the possibility that this might occur at some specific locations with the proper parameters cannot be eliminated completely, later work has shown that longer durations of stimulation trains are more rewarding than short ones. According to Coleman and Berger (1978): "The relationship between train duration and relative reinforcement strength is described by a monotonically increasing curve over a wide range of values." The stimulation during later periods in a train does not become aversive but is not as rewarding as that occurring at the beginning of the train. Thus, as Rolls (1975) suggests: "Rats terminate brain-stimulation reward so that they can switch it on again [p. 75]." Coleman and Berger have recently used a sophisticated signal-detection procedure to determine the function relating stimulus duration to its rewardingness or "utility." The results fit closely a negatively accelerating power function: Utility $= d^c$, where $d =$ the duration of electrical stimulation and $c =$ a constant ranging from .53 to .79 for different animals. This result (admittedly from only a small number of animals and using only a small range of durations) has strong implications for the rest principle because it supports the one assumption within the principle for which there was no physiological evidence (i.e., that use is necessary before rest in order to produce an increase in the strength of neural connections and that the increment per unit of time is greatest during an early part of the rest period).

This support is dependent on the assumption that self-stimulation reinforces the preceding response because it allows the relevant pathways to rest, either by inhibiting or removing excitation from them. The degree to which the pathways is strengthened is of course the relative reinforcement produced by the ICSS (i.e.

its utility). Coleman and Berger's results then indicate that the increase in strength is greatest during the early part of the rest period (i.e., during the early part of the period when electrical stimulation is being given to neurons inhibiting or removing excitation from the pathway). The strength continues to grow during later parts of the rest period, but the increment per unit time becomes progressively smaller.

Confirmation that the rate of increase in strength is greatest during the early stages of rest also confirms the requirement of use before rest in the rest principle. For instance, imagine a pathway that has been resting for such a long time that the increments per unit of time are nearly zero. Using the pathway again starts a new rest period, during the early stages of which the pathway will increase rapidly in strength. The only way for the pathway to grow during rest is for it to be used first. For all connections that have ever been used before in the life of the organism, having strengthening occur most rapidly when the rest is first imposed is equivalent to having use being needed before rest for reinforcement.

It is unfortunately not possible to derive the exact function for the growth in strength as a function of the duration of rest from the changes in utility with the duration of electrical stimulation. Although the firing rate of the electrically stimulated neurons is probably fixed by the stimulation, the ability of these neurons to inhibit or to remove stimulation from the pathway producing the preceding response probably decreases slightly with continued usage. If this allows any of the neurons in the pathway to fire again it could account for some of the reduction in utility. With the parameters used by Coleman and Berger, that contribution seems to account for only a small part of the change in utility; most of the change is probably caused by the increments in strength of the pathway being greatest during the initial portions of the rest period. Nevertheless, because the relative portions of the change produced by the two factors are unknown, one cannot calculate the function of growth versus rest duration.

In closing this chapter, we consider briefly what predictions the *use principle* would make about these forms of learning. Admittedly, I speak about the use principle alone, without added assumptions. Some of the discrepancies discussed might be removed with the proper additional assumptions, but it should be noted that all of the predictions that have been made from the rest principle in the preceding pages have been based upon the principle itself without modification.

The use principle would predict that the least likely response to be learned when a strong physiological need or some other intense stimulus is present is the response that reduces the drive or stimulus. If a hungry animal makes a response that does not reduce hunger, the stimulation from hunger remains, and the response can be emitted repeatedly, becoming stronger with each repetition. The response that produces food and thus eventually removes hunger could only be made once during each hunger–satiety cycle: It drastically changes the stimulus situation and removes the primary stimulus (hunger); consequently, the pathway from hunger to the response could not be used again until the physiological need had reappeared.

Similarly, when a strong external stimulus such as electric shock is present, the animal would be most likely to learn responses that further intensified the stimulus. Suppose shock, S_E, initially elicited response, R_X. If R_X terminated S_E, the pathway could be used only once. If R_X did not affect S_E, there is a very good chance S_E–R_X might be used again and thus strengthened, but there is also a chance that some other competitive stimulus might intervene, eliciting its own responses and curtailing the use of S_E–R_X. But if R_X greatly increased the shock intensity, it becomes much less likely that any other stimulus could intervene; consequently, the chances that S_E–R_X could be used again and strengthened would be increased. Therefore, animals would not learn to escape shock but rather to approach it. Running in a maze with a shock gradient would be thus toward the end with the highest intensity. Animals would not only approach a fire but would climb into it. Similarly, they would not learn to avoid situations in which intense stimulation is likely but would learn to make responses that would assure that such situations were produced.

The use principle could make an animal learn the contingencies of a response but would not change appropriately the probability that the animal would make that response. If an S_X–R_X pathway produced a response that delivered food and if reverberation within S_X–R_X was still present when the food-related stimuli were received, the simultaneous firing of the units would cause strengthening of S_X–S_{h+food}, S_{h+food}–S_X, and S_{h+food}–R_X, but it would cause no more strengthening of S_X–R_X than would occur if other equally intense stimulus (e.g., S_E) were presented.

In the ICSS studies in which it seemed at first that animals were working to increase hunger or other drives, there would have been no paradox for the use principle. This is exactly what it would predict should happen. The paradox for the use principle was that animals under normal conditions worked to terminate drives. The use principle, however, could also account for animals seeking stimulation of neurons that normally responded to the combination of hunger plus food, if these neurons were also firing before the response was made. It, therefore, would predict properly that priming with "free" stimulation would improve learning and that hunger would also improve performance.

The successfulness of the use principle in predicting this stimulation-seeking behavior, in contrast to its universal failure to account for drive-reduction or escape learning, does not detract from the rest principle. As shown in Chapter 8, for lower levels of stimulation the rest principle becomes identical to the use principle, and both are capable of explaining the findings.

8 Instrumental Learning II: Stimulation Seeking, Optimal Levels, and Pleasure

In Chapter 7 we primarily considered intense stimuli: intense internal stimuli related to physiological drives, intense external ones like shock, and ones that became intense because of the connections they developed. Responses that reduced these intense stimuli usually were strengthened, whereas responses that did not reduce them or actually produced the intense stimuli generally were weakened.

Such learning occurs relatively seldom for humans in modern society. We rarely experience intense hunger or thirst, and intense external stimuli are encountered only infrequently. Most of our behavior appears to be directed toward obtaining stimulation rather than reducing it. As a random sample: At the moment I am writing this, my wife is reading, one daughter is watching TV, and the baby is playing with a revolving toy; even the dog is begging to run free outside. It is difficult to see any of these behaviors as drive or stimulation reducing, but nevertheless it is very likely that all three people would be willing to work or learn some response in order to enter into their stimulation-gathering activities, and the dog has learned previously to open various types of doors and to chew through ropes in order to run free.

In the laboratory, experiments have shown under more controlled circumstances that animals will learn to perform tasks for such rewards as having the light turned on, being allowed to see some particular scene, or obtaining the opportunity to run in an activity wheel (Barnes & Kish, 1958; Butler, 1953, 1958; Butler & Harlow, 1954; Harwitz, 1956; Kish, 1955; Premack, 1962; Premack, Collier, & Roberts, 1957; Roberts et al., 1958). These are, of course, the results that could not be dealt with adequately by traditional drive-reduction theories and led to postulations of drives for seeing, running, arousal, and so on and then to other drives for turning off the stimuli. The circularity of this approach has been mentioned earlier.

In contrast, the *rest principle* automatically predicts the occurrence of such stimulation-seeking behavior. The prediction comes from the assumption within the principle that connections are strengthened most rapidly during the early parts of the rest period. Evidence in favor of this assumption from ICSS studies was discussed in Chapter 7. Although, as stated at that time, there was no direct physiological evidence for this assumption, there is suggestive evidence from the physiological studies. With denervation supersensitivity, a stage eventually is reached after which no further increases in sensitivity develop with further rest (e.g., Roper, 1976). It seems likely that other processes with shorter time courses, such as those regulating transmitter release, also reach such a stage; the alternative, that the amount of transmitter released per action potential continues increasing indefinitely, seems impossible—a limit eventually must be reached even if it is only when every molecule of transmitter within the synaptic ending is released with a single firing. Unfortunately, the studies on the short-term processes generally have been concerned with the reduction occurring during use and not specifically with the recovery rate during rest; findings during the early stages after denervation are confounded by the initial flood of transmitter; and the findings from receptor blackade studies are confounded during the early stages of rest by the continued presence of the blocking agent. Thus the present physiological evidence, although generally supporting this assumption, provides little basis for concluding what the time course is. We therefore, are forced to rely upon the data from the ICSS studies.

If we assume that the strength of a connection grows as some negatively accelerating function of the duration of rest, such as Coleman and Berger's power function (1978, see Chapter 7, this volume) and that the initial firing causes some weakening (or some latency is involved in starting the strengthening), the connection grows most rapidly if it is used at some optimal rate, r_{opt}, that is, once every t_{opt} time units, where t_{opt} is determined by the tangent (- - -) to the curve from the initial starting point in Fig. 8.1.

If the firing rate is faster than r_{max} so that the time between uses is less than t_{max}, the connection will become weaker. If the interval between uses is greater than t_{max}, but less than t_{opt}, the connection will become stronger, but not as rapidly as it does if used only once every t_{opt} time units. Similarly, if the interval is longer than t_{opt}, the connection will become stronger, but again not as rapidly as if it were used at intervals of t_{opt}.

Figure 8.1 can be redrawn to show the rate of change in the strength of a connection as a function of the rate of use (Fig. 8.2). This is approximately the same as Fig. 5.11 introduced earlier (p. 59). For reasons discussed at the end of the chapter, this is called a *Wundtian curve*.

This graphic derivation of the Wundtian curve is relatively general, but the result nevertheless has been checked with computer simulations of various rest

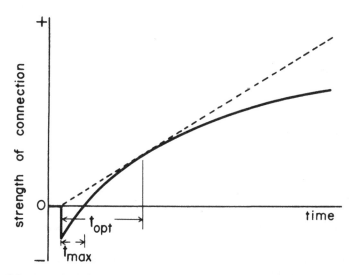

FIG. 8.1.   The growth of a connection as a function of the duration of rest. In the figure, some weakening occurs because of the initial use, which is consistent (but not necessary) for the assumption that use alone weakens. The maximal increase in strength follows the dashed line (---) and occurs if the connection is used once every t_{opt} time units. It is quite possible that the physiological processes involved in strengthening have some latency for starting after the connection is used. In that case the curve would have an S shape conforming to the negatively accelerating curve only after some delay. There would still be an optimal rate of firing, r_{opt}, for strengthening connections if both the weakening after one use and the latency for the beginning of strengthening occurred or if either of these occurred. If there is a latency, optimal levels of firing would still be produced by forms of the rest principle in which only rapid repetitive use causes weakening.

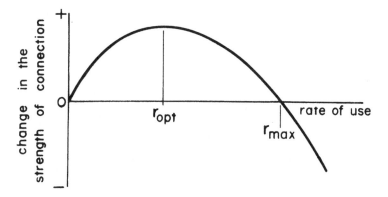

FIG. 8.2.   The change in the strength of a connection as a function of the rate of use. $r_{opt} = t_{opt}^{-1}$ from Fig. 8.1; $r_{max} = t_{max}^{-1}$.

principle models. For instance, in one it was assumed that the strength of a given connection could be altered only in discrete steps all the same size, but the probability, p, that a given connection would be strengthened was highest early in the rest period: $p = e^{-m}$, where m is the number of time cycles since the connection was last used. Whenever it was used, its strength was lowered by one unit, or in another variation the probability of weakening was e^{-1}. In another simulation the changes in strength for a given connection were assumed to be continuous rather than discrete, and the amount of both weakening if used again and strengthening when resting was assumed to vary with the interval following the last use: Both followed a negative exponential curve, e^{-cm}, but the constant c was larger for the weakening, so it had a shorter time course. In all the simulations, Wundtian curves similar to that in Fig. 8.2 were produced.

Before considering how the Wundtian curve helps to account for stimulus-seeking behavior, I would like to mention a possible additional assumption that modifies the curve slightly. The assumption is that there is a slow continual degrading of connections occurring independently of the changes caused by the rest principle. This "additional assumption" is not part of the rest principle and whether it is correct or not has little bearing on the present theory; nevertheless, it does complement the rest principle and helps to explain a few phenomena. I specifically identify any conclusions that require this additional assumption.

If the additional assumption is applied to Fig. 8.2, it raises the values along the ordinate, so that there is a decrease in the strength of connections with a zero rate of use. (Compare Fig. 5.11, which incorporates the additional assumption, with Fig. 8.2, which does not.) A minimum rate, r_{min}, is then needed just to maintain the strength; to paraphrase the Red Queen: "With the 'additional assumption' you have to run (at a speed of r_{min}) just to stay where you are." Consequently, forgetting could occur because of a weakening of connections that were not used often enough rather than as a result only of interference.

The Wundtian curve generated by the rest principle (regardless of whether the addition assumption is included) can be used to show how responses are reinforced when they bring the firing rate closer to r_{opt}, either by decreasing overly high rates of firing (as covered in the preceding chapter) or by increasing overly low rates.

We consider an S neuron (or neurons) whose firing rate can be varied by external circumstances. Responses can be divided into two classes: (1) those elicited by outputs from S; and (2) those elicited independently of S by outputs from other, O, neurons. I first examine the former and show how S–R connecting producing responses that increase the firing rate of S are preferentially strengthened. Imagine two responses elicited by S: R_1 does not increase the rate of firing of S, whereas R_2 does (e.g., approaching a dim light). As shown in Fig. 8.3, after a period of using S–R_1 the connections will have been increased in strength by less than 3 units, because the average rate of use of the pathway was at the low level produced by the initial value for S. In contrast, since R_2

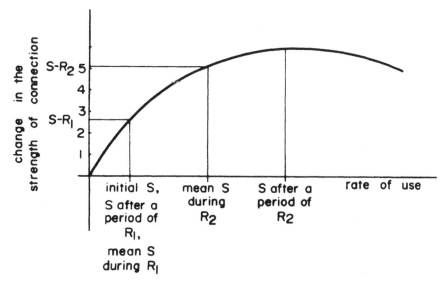

FIG. 8.3. A portion of the Wundtian curve from Fig. 8.2, showing why a response elicited by S that increases the firing rate of S toward r_{opt} is reinforced more than a response that does not increase S.

progressively increases the firing rate of S, the rate of firing of the S-R_2 pathway also will increase progressively during a period of making response R_2. The net increase in the strength of S-R_2 will be determined by the mean rate of firing of the pathway during the period of use that is approximately half of the sum of the initial plus final firing rates and, as shown in the figure, amounts to about 5 arbitrary units.

Another factor that would contribute to the greater reinforcement of R_2 is the greater ability of S with an increased firing rate to compete with other neurons for the domination of behavior. Consequently, S-R_2 is likely to continue being used longer before being interrupted by some other activity and thus will show more strengthening than S-R_1. A response elicited by S that terminated S would receive the least reinforcement because it could be used only once.

The means by which near-optimum firing of S reinforces responses elicited by other, O, neurons is a bit more complicated. The paradigm considered is: O elicits R, which causes S to begin firing at a rate close to r_{opt}. The direct O-R pathway receives little strengthening because it is used only briefly on each trial. The reinforcement comes about primarily because of the growth of O-S and S-O connections. When R indirectly makes S fire because of external circumstances, any output from the preceding firing of O, R, or the O-R pathway to S, from reverberations in the O-R pathway to S, or from the continued presence of O to S will be able to contribute to the already assured firing of S, and because of this use these connections to S become stronger. The joint presence of O firing and S firing also may start reverberation between the two on any pathways not blocked by inhibition; the reverberation will strengthen S–O connections as well as O–S connections. Consequently, in the future O will cause partial activation of the S units and will have a larger reverberatory field, which will help O to dominate competing neurons. On subsequent trials, connections from the additional neurons activated by O to R also will be strengthened by use, thus providing multiple pathways by which O can elicit R. This strengthening of course works best if S is made to fire at r_{opt}; if S fires at a rate much slower than r_{opt}, there will be less use of the connections between O and S and less strengthening; if S is made to fire faster than R_{max} we have a punishment paradigm and the preceding response may be weakened. (With the exception of this last comment about rates above r_{max}, all the preceding arguments are identical to those employed in *use principle* theories [e.g., Hebb, 1949], for the simple reason that at low rates of firing the rest principle is equivalent to the use principle.)

The Wundtian curve relating the strengthening of connections to the rate of use (Fig. 8.2) thus translates to being a curve relating the amount of reinforcement of preceding responses produced by different rates of use, either within the pathway producing the response or in independent pathways. In other words, there is an optimal rate of use for reinforcing responses. This process would work for all kinds of neurons. The S units could represent neurons firing in proportion to stimulus intensity, neurons fired by output from a multitude of specific feature analyzers (that are themselves stimulated by particular characteristics in the external stimuli [i.e., the information content]), neurons fired by output from neurons sensitive only to changes in stimuli (e.g., ones that fire primarily when light is first turned on or off), or even neurons generally stimulated by excitation in motor response pathways. Although this involves an oversimplification, these results could be used to predict Wundtian curves relating all these factors to reinforcement. Consequently, optimal levels of stimulus intensity (Leuba, 1955), information flow from the environment (Glanzer, 1958), stimulus complexity (Dember & Earl, 1957), stimulus change (McClelland et al., 1953), and motor activity (Premack, 1962) would occur for reinforcing preceding responses.

One problem with these conclusions is that they often require the postulating of converging networks, for instance, from all feature analyzers to neurons whose firing rate would then be determined by the information flow in the external stimuli. Without such networks, the information content would be represented only by the number of neurons activated and not by the rate of firing of any one neuron. A similar problem is that this analysis neglects the fact that stimulus intensity may be encoded as either the frequency of firing or the number of neurons activated (Mountcastle, 1967) (i.e., with low-intensity stimuli firing only neurons with low thresholds, whereas high-intensity stimuli fire both low and high threshold neurons). Evidence for such a relationship at the central level may be seen in EEG records and more recently in the studies on the cortical blood flow: High-intensity stimuli cause widespread increases in blood flow throughout the cortex, apparently reflecting widespread activation of a very large number of neurons (Lassen et al., 1978; Maximillian et al., 1977). Finally, the foregoing analysis neglects the temporal properties of the stimuli, except for their effect on change-sensitive neurons. Consequently, it is not able to account for the aversiveness of monotonous weak stimulation.

A more complicated analysis that includes the factors neglected in the simple analysis shows how similar conclusions regarding optimal levels are generated by the rest principle without postulating converging networks. It also accounts for various results that the simple analysis could not.

I start with the effects of encoding intensity as the number of neurons firing, which have been examined in a computer simulation. In this simulation, 100 stimulation-sensitive S neurons were assumed to have normally distributed thresholds, so that the number firing for various stimulus intensities formed an ogive curve (Fig. 8.4). Each S neuron was assumed to have random connections to other neurons, thus leading to possible responses and also back onto other S neurons. Therefore, the firing of the S neurons is an internal stimulus for eliciting more firing in the S neurons; in other words, reverberation can occur. The relationship between the number of S neurons fired by the initial momentary presentation of the external stimulus and the subsequent firing caused by reverberation is assumed to be linear (the straight line in Fig. 8.4). For instance, an external stimulus with an intensity of 9 arbitrary units fires 77 of the S neurons. The firing of 77 neurons then produces a reverberation input equivalent to an external stimulus with an intensity of 7.8 units, according to the straight line, which in turn fires 64 of the S neurons, etc. Thus the reverberation rapidly runs down and, in the example in the figure, stops after 4 cycles.

In the figure, the thresholds are shown as remaining constant, but in the simulation the thresholds changed as the strength of the connections changed, in accordance with the rest principle. Consequently, if the ogive curve is started far to the right of the straight line (i.e., high thresholds) and very long times (effectively infinite) are allowed between stimulus presentations, experience with momentary stimuli of a variety of intensities causes the ogive to shift to the left until it overlaps the straight line. The ogival shape, however, is generally maintained.

The relationship found in these simulations between the stimulus intensity and the sum of the amount of strengthening minus the weakening of connections (i.e., the net change in the strength of connections) followed a Wundtian curve, like that shown in Fig. 8.2. Low-intensity stimuli excited only a few neurons, which were then allowed to rest, resulting in a small increase in strength. As intensity increased, the number of neurons being excited increased, thus raising the number of connections with the potential of being strengthened; at the same time, however, the number being used repeatedly because of reverberation began to increase. For increases from very low to moderate intensities, the former

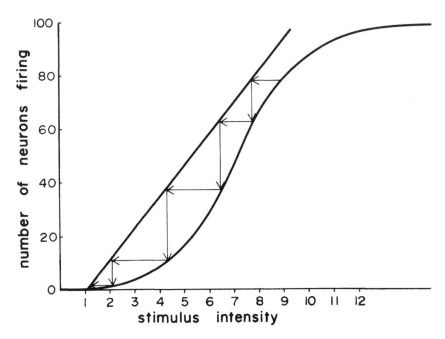

FIG. 8.4.   Production of reverberation after momentary application of an external
stimulus. The ogive curve represents the number of S neurons fired by different
intensities of stimulation. The straight diagonal line represents the equivalent
intensity produced by different numbers of S neurons firing back upon other S
neurons. The arrows show the course of reverberation caused by momentarily
presenting an external stimulus with an intensity of 9. The stimulus itself fires 77
neurons. Returning feedback from these 77 excites 64; the 64 excite 37; the 37
excite 10; and the 10 excite 1. Changes in threshold caused by use and rest during
the course of the reverberation are not shown but were included in the computer
simulation.

factor prevailed, and the net increase in strength increased. Eventually, with
stronger intensities, the number being used repeatedly began to predominate,
thus reducing the net increase in strength.

A strange thing happened when the ogive curve had shifted so that it overlap-
ped the straight line: For stimuli more intense than the lower crossover point, the
first reverberation fired more neurons than the initial stimulus, and the second
reverberation fired more than the first. The firing only subsided when the connections had been weakened sufficiently by continual use. Under these conditions
there often was a net decrease in the strength of connection, and the ogive would
shift toward the right. The general relationship between intensity and net change
in strength still followed a Wundtian curve, but with an abrupt decrease occurring as intensity increased beyond the crossover point.

Next I examined what happened if the stimulus was applied for long periods of time rather than just momentarily. The reverberation from the first external input added to the input from the continued presence of the stimulus. The result was that even weak external stimuli produced a net decrease in strength of connections if applied long enough. In effect, the equivalent intensity of a stimulus was a function of the external intensity times the duration that it was applied. A family of curves then related the net change in the strength of connections to duration and intensity. For shorter duration, Wundtian curves related the strength change to intensity, but for longer durations the Wundtian curves shifted to the left until eventually all intensities produced weakening—with stronger intensities producing more weakening than weak ones. For low intensities, Wundtian curves also related the strength change to duration, but for high intensities all duration produced weakening.

Therefore, the previously discussed conclusions about optimal levels still hold for briefly applied external stimuli, but there are different conclusions for longer durations of stimulation. Because the optimal point shifts to the left and eventually disappears with increases in duration, responses that stop the presentation of monotonous stimuli are strengthened. One class of such responses is eye movements, which are discussed a little later. Another way to decrease the firing caused by monotonous stimuli is to have some other stimulus appear and have attention directed to it. Attention is covered in detail in Chapter 10, but what is important for the present discussion is that attention somehow inhibits activity in unattended channels and modalities, as demonstrated in both behavioral and electrophysiological studies (Hernández-Péon, Scherrer, & Jouvet, 1956). Consequently, as long as attention is focused on other matters, a low-intensity continuous stimulus may not even be represented at central levels, and a response for physically turning it off will not be produced. As a simple example, the buzz of our aquarium pump is not generally heard during the day and is certainly not bothersome, but someone trying to sleep in the same room with it will find it very loud and annoying and, if given the chance, will try to turn it off. To compound the problem, when competing stimuli are missing, the monotonous stimulus itself attracts attention and prevents thinking or daydreaming; thus it seems that the aversiveness is caused partly by the prolonged overuse of the neurons stimulated by the buzz plus the reduction of firing in other areas to far below r_{opt}. This latter aspect may be particularly important in the negative reinforcing properties of prolonged intermittent stimulation, as with a dripping water faucet or the classic water torture.

Looking at the other side of this issue, stimuli that momentarily attract attention should be reinforcing to the extent that they inhibit overuse of pathways stimulated by monotonous input and increase firing in underused pathways. The most reinforcing stimuli would be ones with sufficient intensity or intrinsic importance to capture attention but not so strong as to cause too much reverberation. They should hold attention long enough to assure that a large number of neurons are used and sufficient rest given to any neurons having been fired by monotonous input but not so long that many are fired repeatedly. The complexity should be high enough that rarely excited feature analyzers are fired but not so high that attention is captured for too long a time.

Let us look a bit closer at these feature analyzers, which have been mentioned in passing earlier, and at the pathways leading to them. Sensory input systems appear to be organized in a hierarchical manner. The lower-order neurons receiving the stimulus input first are sensitive to very general characteristics: in the visual system, for instance, to the presence of light within a broad range of wavelengths on their retinal fields. At slightly higher levels there are neurons that are more selective and are fired, for instance, only by the onset or termination of light, by light on their retinal field when and only when the surrounding fields are not illuminated, or by very narrow bands of wavelengths. Next come neurons fired only by lines or edges in the visual stimulus with particular orientations, by movement of stimuli, and by movement of only lines with particular orientations. Eventually, at the top of the hierarchical pyramids, are neurons sensitive to very specific features only (e.g., Rolls' [1975] white-syringe-plus-hunger neuron, or the hand-detector visual neuron found by Gross, Rocha-Miranda, and Bender [1972]). Some inversions occur, with higher order neurons being less specific than lower ones (e.g., the higher one may respond to a configuration appearing anywhere in the visual field, whereas the lower one responds to the configuration only in a particular retinal field), but as a general rule the higher order neurons are more selective and therefore are activated less frequently.

It seems very likely that such hierarchical pyramids are found not only in the sensory systems but are common throughout the nervous system, and also that the sensory ones have projections to more plastic parts of the brain, as evidenced by the feature analyzer Rolls found in the hypothalamus.

When a simple familiar stimulus is presented (e.g., an easily recognized picture of a hand), very little firing is needed at the lower levels of the pyramid to cause the top "hand-detector" neuron to fire. A more complex picture (e.g., a hand holding an apple) will cause more of the infrequently used top neurons to fire (hand and apple detectors). Inasmuch as any use of rarely activated connections is reinforcing, two top neurons firing will cause more reinforcement than just one. Recognizing two objects from the same stimulus will, however, require a slightly longer duration of stimulation to the lower-order neurons used in both the "hand" pyramid and the "apple" pyramid. As long as the duration is still in the flat part of the Wundtian curve relating duration to the strengthening of connections, this will not subtract much from the gain in reinforcement produced by having two top neurons fired; it could even add to it if the duration required to fire the hand detector alone was well below the optimal point on the Wundtian curve. Therefore, as complexity increases from low to moderate levels, there will be a net gain in the reinforcing effect. At still higher levels of complexity, however, the duration of use of the lower-order neurons will reach the sharply declining portions of the Wundtian curve, and this will offset the gains produced by having more top neurons firing; consequently, there will be a net decrease in the reinforcement.

Adding to this relationship will be the effects of rest imposed on other neurons while the visual stimulus is being attended. This will depend on the preceding overall level of activation, but, in general, short durations of rest will be more beneficial than long ones. With very complex figures, which require prolonged attention, the resulting suppression of the firing rate elsewhere below r_{opt} will contribute to the relative decrease in reinforcement. Perhaps these relationships might be clearer if we imagine how they might be translated into the accompanying emotional responses. A subject who has been observing a very complex figure for a long time might be found saying, "I don't care what else is in the picture; I don't want to look at it any more" (i.e., the negative factors from overuse of the lower-order "looking" neurons are greater than the positive factors from firing top "feature" neurons). "I'm tired of it and want to do something else" (i.e., negative factors from the suppression of firing elsewhere, which are experienced as boredom, have become strong).

The relationship between complexity and the reinforcing potential, therefore, will itself be a Wundtian curve, with an optimal level of complexity occurring at some intermediate level in line with Dember and Earl's earlier suggestions (1957). Notice that this occurs without having to postulate a converging network from the hand detector, apple detector, etc. onto a general "information-flow" neuron. Of course, if such a network does exist, the prolonged use of this information-flow neuron with very complex stimuli would contribute to the reduction in the reinforcing effect, and in general the converging network would improve the efficiency of these processes.

In the previous example, it was assumed that the stimuli were familiar and easily recognized; in other words, the particular pattern of excitation imposed on the lower-order neurons led almost immediately to the firing of the top neurons. If the pattern is somewhat ambiguous or less familiar, however, traveling the route with the strongest connections in the pyramid will not complete successfully the analysis of the stimulus, and routes with progressively weaker connection will be traversed ("No, it's not a dog—the back slants downward—Aha! it's a hyena.") until a top neuron is fired that properly covers all the lower-order features.

It might be mentioned that the rest principle allows both the storage of a large amount of memory within the same pyramid and the search through progressively weaker routes within the pyramid. The continued use of the strongest ("dog") pathway quickly weakens these connections, so that the next-to-strongest connections from the same lower-order neurons will be traversed. This does not exclude, however, control of the activity from outside the pyramid (e.g., by keeping attention focused on the stimulus or particular aspects of the stimulus or by biasing one possible route over others).

If the duration for properly analyzing the stimulus is not too long, the firing of the weaker connections and the eventual use of an extremely rarely used top neuron ("hyena" rather than just "dog") will increase the reinforcing effect. As before with complexity, however, if very long times are required to complete the analysis, the prolonged use of the lower-order neurons eventually will reduce the net reinforcement. Consequently, the relationship between novelty (or ambiguity) and reinforcement will follow a Wundtian curve. An interaction between familiarity and complexity would also be predicted. If the routes in the pyramids are well-developed and require less time to make the top neurons fire, the Wundtian curve for complexity would be shifted to the right and the greatest reinforcement would come from more complex stimuli. An artist might enjoy more complexity in a painting than a young child does. Of course, the artist would also enjoy more novelty and ambiguity. Similarly, a young child might prefer a book of dog pictures; an older child, a book of less familiar African animals; and the zoologist, a book showing various rare strains of subtly differing African animals.

The previous examples have assumed that the subject has control over the time spent attending the stimulus. If the stimuli are instead presented to the subject for only a certain period of time, the optimal reinforcement would be produced if the presentation time was just long enough for each stimulus to be analyzed and the top neuron fired a few times. An overly fast rate of presentation in which the bottom neurons are able to fire but not enough time is given for allowing the top neurons to fire would be particularly aversive. The time needed for properly analyzing a stimulus depends, of course, on the prior learning experience of the individual. It is most exasperating to listen to a lecture presented in a language you understand only partially: You hear most of the words, but there is not time enough to catch the ideas being presented. The same lecture may be quite enjoyable to people well-versed in the language; to people knowing none of the language or related languages, the lecture would be equivalent to the buzz of the aquarium pump (i.e., aversive only if other stimuli are not present to attract attention).

Situations in which we have a good control over the rate of stimulation will be very reinforcing and enjoyable. I think much of the pleasure most people feel from driving their own cars on the open road comes from the high degree of control they have over stimulation input from various sensory modalities and motion detectors and over the flow of information. For more stimulation, the driver needs only to accelerate to a higher speed. Furthermore, the speed chosen should be a function of the inherent stimulation from the particular highway: Higher rates of speed will be chosen, if possible, on an expressway where the stimulus objects are far away from the road and therefore produce less stimulation particularly of motion detectors, where there is a low density of interesting (information) features, and where practically no activity is needed to drive the car. In fact, an argument could be made in favor of displaying advertising billboards close to the highway, because these should reduce the speed drivers would choose. The anger produced by traffic jams can be seen as being caused largely by frustration from the lack of expected reinforcement, because the driver can no longer choose his own rate of stimulation.

An important way of controlling visual stimulation is through eye movements. There are several different types of eye movements. There are the very small "nystagmus" movements occurring 30 to 70 times per second. When a stationary point stimulus is viewed, nystagmus keeps the point stimulating different receptors in the fovea of the retina. If the target begins moving, small movements occur that track the stimulus, tending to bring it back toward the fovea but usually lagging slightly behind the stimulus. If a new stimulus appears in the periphery, a rapid large "saccade" movement is made, bringing the stimulus into the fovea region. This is called the *fixation reflex*. Saccades also are made to bring a target back into the fovea if the nystagmus movements have caused it to drift out.

Eye movements can be controlled voluntarily, by reflexes from inputs from head and body movements, by stimuli from the inner ear, and by proprioceptive feedback from receptors in the eye muscles (Fiorentini & Maffei, 1977). However, I discuss here primarily the control from the visual system itself.

Each of these eye movements causes the visual stimulation that just preceded it to be terminated. Therefore, the connections from the visually stimulated neurons to the neurons triggering the eye movements could be learned according to the rest principle (if the connections were formed by genetic guidance, the rest principle assures that they would not be weakened but rather strengthened.). It is also true that each of the movements causes an increased firing in pathways that were not used previously, and this could add to the strengthening of the connections triggering them.

Let us consider first the fixation reflex. A recent analysis of the types of neurons in the parietal lobe of monkeys (Yin & Mountcastle, 1977) has shown one class of neurons stimulated by visual input to the periphery of the retina but not by stimulation of the fovea. A response that could, therefore, terminate the firing of these neurons in general would be a saccade that positioned the light stimulus in the fovea. Yin and Mountcastle also located another class of cells that fired only when such saccades were made (and therefore probably were involved in producing the response) and a third class that fired both to the peripheral visual stimulation and during the production of the saccade (and therefore probably represents a link between the visual-input- stimulated neurons and the neurons triggering the saccade). It is true that a saccade to some other peripheral location outside the field of one particular neuron of the first class initially activated by the stimulus also would suppress its firing. However, even the fields found in an adult animal are large and overlapping. Consequently, the only response likely to eliminate firing in all the neurons initially stimulated would be a saccade to the fovea. The gradient of firing found, with the higher rates elicited by stimuli farthest from the fovea, also could help direct the saccade toward the fovea as well as eventually control the magnitude of the saccade needed to position the stimulus in the fovea. Of course, the animal could also terminate stimulation by closing its eyes. This reponse would not, however, be as advantageous as a saccade to the fovea: The saccade not only terminates its own stimulus but also causes stimulation of the previously unexcited foveal region that closing the eyes would not cause.

Next let us consider the nystagmus produced to a stationary target. If the effects of these motions are eliminated, for instance, by the use of a small projector mounted on a contact lens that moves with the eye and thus produces stabilized retinal images, perception of the stimulus disappears in a few seconds. This rapid disappearance of perception demonstrates that at some point or points in the pathways leading to perception the firing rates are too rapid (i.e., far above r_{max}). This then is in agreement with the results from the computer simulation in which prolonged stimulation even with weak stimuli caused a weakening of connections. A small eye movement, however, can shift the stimulus on the retina under normal conditions, and for any patterned stimulus there is a good chance that many of the areas previously illuminated will now be in the dark. Consequently, "on" firing elicited from these areas by the initial position of the stimulus will be terminated and the neurons will be forced to rest by inhibition from the competitive "off" responses now occurring. Similarly, many of the areas previously in the dark will now receive light, and therefore the previous "off" responses will be terminated and the neurons making them will be forced to rest by the "on" responses now being produced. Connections from these pathways, fired by the initial position but not by the new position, to the neurons that trigger the nystagmus would be allowed to rest after use and would grow stronger.

If a point target begins moving, motion detectors are stimulated. The response that would terminate this firing is an eye movement that tracks the moving stimulus, thus reducing the movement of the stimulus across the retina. Consequently, connections from motion detectors to the neurons triggering the appropriate tracking nystagmus would be strengthened, and a moving target would elicit tracking, as has been found (Cohen, Matsuo, & Raphan, 1977).

If the visual system is viewed as a hierarchical pyramid, as previously discussed, the net effect of all these eye movements is to decrease the firing of the bottom neurons that otherwise would have an overly high firing rate, while increasing the firing of the less frequently used top neurons. Each movement terminates the lower-order stimulation that elicits it (excitation of peripheral receptors, of fovea receptors, or of motion detectors) but at the same time keeps stimuli positioned in the area of the retina with the greatest representation in the cortex (i.e., the fovea) and prevents habituation of the lower-order neurons, thus allowing us to have continual visual perception at the central level. It seems likely that the connections involved in eliciting the eye movements as a result of visual input are strengthened primarily by the rest allowed the bottom neurons, but the increased firing of the top neurons could also contribute to their production. The firing of the top neurons might be particularly important in reinforcing eye movements directed by attention and those under voluntary control.

In general, we have no similar peripheral mechanisms for terminating persistent inputs in other sensory modalities. There are, however, neuronal pathways to the inner ear that lower sensitivity when loud noises are present. Animals drinking strong unpleasantly flavored solutions will adopt response patterns that minimize contact between the solution and the tongue. In the presence of unpleasant odors, sniffing is suppressed and breathing becomes very shallow. And of course there are responses such as moving off a tack, holding one's nose, or covering the ears. Selective attention, as mentioned earlier, can also inhibit firing in unattended pathways. In the visual system, people can attend selectively to certain kinds of targets or parts of the visual array even in the absence of eye movements (Sperling & Melchner, 1978); in the auditory system, people can attend to the message presented to one ear and thus prevent the message presented to the other from reaching awareness. Another method for helping to prevent habituation in sensory systems would be the use of redundant input pathways linked by lateral inhibition. The pathway with the highest firing rate or lowest threshold would initially inhibit other pathways excited by the same stimulus. After the first pathway has weakened, the next in strength will take up the job of signaling the presence of the stimulus, inhibiting the first in the process and thus allowing it to regain its strength. Such redundant pathways appear to be employed, at least on the output side, for maintaining tonic excitation of muscles. The job is shared by numerous neurons and muscle fibers so that no one neuron or fiber will be used too often. Such temporal sharing can occur automatically in a system operating with the negative feedback of the rest principle but would be very difficult to have in a system built with the use principle.

Several cases have been mentioned so far in which the reinforcing effect came not from a single source but from the combined actions of neurons (e.g., in different modalities or at different levels in the hierarchy of pyramids). The effects can be cooperative, as when eye movements are reinforced both by reduced firing in lower-order neurons and increased firing in higher-order ones. In other cases the effects may counteract one another. For instance, a stimulus with an optimal level of complexity and novelty but with a very high physical intensity would produce positively reinforcing effects from the higher-order neurons but negatively reinforcing effects from the intensity-sensitive lower-order neurons.

Cooperative effects also could play a role in drive-reduction learning. When a hungry animal is given a pleasant-tasting food after, for instance, bar pressing, the response will be reinforced by the rest given to the neurons in the $S\text{-}R_{BP}$

pathway, with the help of classical conditioning of the connections to the S_{h+food} $-R_{in}$ pathway, as discussed in Chapter 7. At the same time, however, perhaps in other parts of the brain, infrequently used top neurons are being fired: neurons that represent specific features of the environment, the bar-pressing response, and the food stimuli. The strengthening of these connections, which requires no externally imposed rest, would then contribute to the memory of the events. Of course, some top neurons nearly always are being used and connections are being strengthened regardless of whether food is obtained or not. When the animal made incorrect responses this also was being recorded. There may be factors associated with obtaining and eating food that enhance memory storage, as discussed later (p. 189), but the important difference between the memories stored after successful and unsuccessful responses is only that the former include connections to food-stimuli neurons. Consequently, in the future the stimuli associated with bar pressing will elicit food-stimulated top neurons, what might be called anticipation of food. As mentioned in the criticism of the use principle in Chapter 7, this will not make the animal press the bar again; it could, however, help the stimuli associated with the bar gain dominance over other stimuli and thus be more likely to control the behavior. In addition, on subsequent trials when the stimuli from the bar elicit anticipatory firing of food-stimuli neurons, the connections from these additional neurons to R_{BP} would grow stronger when factors discussed in Chapter 7 make the animal press the bar, thus giving multiple pathways for the production of the response. The possibility that the cerebral cortex represents the primary location for these top neurons is discussed in Chapter 9.

It should be mentioned that failure to give food when the bar is pressed will cause rapid weakening only of the S-R_{BP} pathways discussed in Chapter 7. The connections developed between top neurons are nearly impossible to weaken under normal circumstances because top neurons can be used only infrequently; the development of new connections could cause interference, and if the "additional assumption" is employed, they would be weakened by prolonged disuse but otherwise remain intact. To the extent that these top neurons become important for influencing behavior, it will become necessary for animals to develop a special mechanism for counteracting them in order for extinction to occur rapidly. The hippocampus (Chapter 9) might provide this mechanism.

I discuss later in greater detail this memory storage for food procurement events and how eating could enhance it, but as an introduction let us consider human verbal memory storage. It has been found that a very important characteristic determining whether a word in a list will be remembered is the ease with which it can be imaged (i.e., the extent to which it evokes a picture in our minds). Some unpublished work I once did suggested that the ease of imaging was also important for remembering abstract sounds. Conversely, the ability to remember abstract diagrams was strongly influenced by the ease with which the subjects developed names or descriptive words for them. It might also be mentioned that the major trick involved in most mnemonic systems (i.e., methods for improving one's memory) is imagining a visual representation of verbal input. One tries to form pictures connecting adjacent items in a list of words, or of the words with "hook" words that already have been memorized. The benefit to memory derived from visualizing verbal stimuli, or verbalizing visual ones, could be caused merely by the greater attention used, the longer time spent concentrating on the stimuli, or the fact that they become represented in two ways in memory rather than in just one. These explanations, however, do not seem completely satisfactory. Spending additional time and effort trying to memorize words can be beneficial, but not so beneficial as spending the time visualizing the words, and I doubt if spending the time thinking of synonyms and thus double representation in memory would be as useful.

I would like to suggest the possibility that there are mutually inhibitory arrangements between the different memory systems so that selective attention to one suppresses firing in the others. When one tries picturing a word, the activity in the verbal system is inhibited and, conversely, when the attention is focused on the verbal system, firing in the visual system is curtailed. The inhibition of a system after it has been used would prevent reverberation and strengthen the previously activated pathways. This might not help particularly the connections at the top of a pyramid, but it would be beneficial to all connections also used in other pyramids. When the use of a pyramid is followed by use of other pyramids in the same modality, only the connections used solely by the first pyramid are allowed to rest after firing and become stronger. Merely switching to another modality would be beneficial, but active inhibition would also suppress any spontaneous firing in the first pyramid.

To use an example from the typical instructions for using mnemonics systems: Suppose a small woman introduces herself to you as Ann Smith. You imagine a picture of the frail creature swinging a huge hammer over an anvil in a smithy. On the anvil is a Queen Anne's lace flower that is about to be smashed by the hammer. The verbal input "Ann Smith" fires and then is inhibited while you form the picture. Then you repeat "Ann Smith, how do you do?" and the verbal activation inhibits the visual system. According to the mnemonic system books, your ability to remember her name will be far greater than if you had merely repeated "Ann Smith" to yourself several times.

Figure 8.5 represents such events schematically. There are various ways in which the sequential use of the two memory systems, A and B, could be produced. In the example of words that are easy to visualize or pictures that are easy to name, the sequential use, which is being postulated as being responsible for the increased ability to remember them, is caused by the nature of the stimuli themselves, essentially because the crossover links between A and B are already strong. In the mnemonics procedures, the sequential use is caused by voluntary control in some way. Sequential use could also be produced by an ongoing response chain, such as that occurring when food is earned and eaten in a Skinner

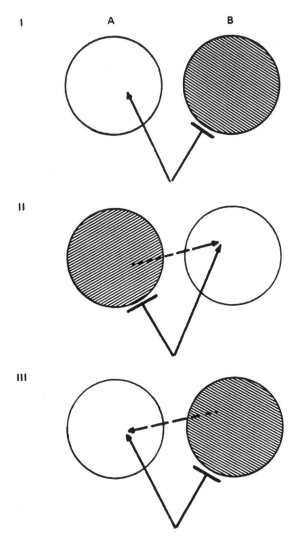

FIG. 8.5. Hypothetical process for particularly effective memory storage with the rest principle. *A* and *B* are two separate neuronal systems, for instance, receiving input primarily from two different sensory modalities. I. Input from some event goes to *A* first; *B* is inhibited, perhaps by the event input, as shown, or by connections between *A* and *B*. II. After a short interval, input from the event goes to *B*, whereas input from the event-stimulated units in *A* arrives in *B* by crossover links, and *A* is inhibited. III. *A* receives input again and *B* is inhibited. The event-stimulated connections in both *A* and *B* are assured of both use and then rest.

box. Attention is first focused on auditory input from the food delivery and then on visual input from the presence of food, on tactual from biting the food, on gustatory from food in the mouth, and on proprioceptive from the act of chewing and swallowing. Consequently, the connections excited by the events in all these modalities and the intermodality associations would be greatly strengthened and a superior memory laid down for these events.

It has been difficult to keep "happiness," "pleasantness," and "unpleasant-ness" out of the discussion so far, and indeed I have not been completely successful in avoiding the use of terms related to these emotional experiences. The concepts are intimately related to reinforcement and the strengthening or weakening of connections. As with other emotions there is the problem of how happiness enters consciousness. Unfortunately, as will be seen, the rest principle does not solve this problem. An interesting relationship does, however, appear. Those situations that the rest principle says should cause a net increase in the strength of connections are also situations in which happiness or pleasure are felt, whereas situations that the principle says should cause a net decrease in the strength of connections cause unhappiness or unpleasantness to be experienced.

The situations mentioned in this and the preceding chapters in which the strength of connections is increasing include: (1) obtaining substances that satisfy a physiological need; (2) obtaining intracranial stimulation to those neurons that normally signal the presence of a substance that reduces drives; (3) escaping or avoiding intense stimulation; (4) obtaining moderate durations of moderate intensity stimulation of various sorts; (5) having attention attracted away from monotonous stimuli by moderate durations of moderate intensity stimulation; (6) having sequential input into various different memory storage systems; and (7) having infrequently used top neurons fired, without overuse of lower-order neurons, because of stimuli with optimal levels of complexity and novelty and an optimal flow of information. The optimal level arguments used for the last situation could be applied also to neurons other than those involved in sensory input. Consequently, moderate levels of physical activity and cognitive activity would cause an increase in the strength of connections. It seems likely that hierarchical pyramids are involved in cognitive activities such as puzzle solving, with the bottom neurons representing the components of the problem. Reaching a solution allows the infrequently used top neurons to be fired without overuse of the bottom neurons and would therefore cause a strengthening of connections.

It can be seen that all the foregoing situations would be classified as pleasura-ble and would increase happiness. For instance, the curve relating the net change in the strength of neuronal connections to the rate of firing (Fig. 8.5) is the same as Wundt (1874) suggested for relating the pleasant–unpleasant continuum to stimulus intensity: This is why I have referred to such curves as "Wundtian curves."

Situations that produced decreases in the strength of connections include: (1) exposure to high-intensity stimuli, including those related to physiological needs;

(2) extinction (e.g., failure to obtain substances that reduce physiological needs when responses are made that previously produced them); (3) long-duration stimulation; (4) with the "additional assumption," prolonged sensory deprivation; and (5) overuse of the bottom neurons of a sensory pyramid without firing the top neurons, as a result of overly high levels of complexity and novelty or an overly high rate of information flow (or, conversely, exposure to random stimulation with no meaning). The last situation can also be extended to cognitive activities, such as puzzles for which no solution can be found, and to cognitive dissonance, in which the bottom neurons would be overused and no easy way found to fire the top neurons. Prolonged overuse of neurons involved in motor activity should also lead to a weakening of connections. All these situations produce unpleasant feelings and unhappiness.

Classical conditioning with an aversive CS such as electric shock may at first appear to contradict this generalization, inasmuch as the UCS–UCR pathway is being strengthened but the situation is unpleasant. It is likely however that, in general, connections are being weakened during such conditioning, and only the connections of neurons within the inhibitory surround of the CS–CR pathway are being strengthened or at least not weakened as much. Consequently, there is a net decrease in the strength of connections in general, which is in agreement with the negative affect. There may, however, be limits as to which connections can influence affect. For instance, conditioning of peripheral reflexes in an organism with a severed spinal column would not directly influence affect, I would imagine, and it is quite possible that changes in the strength of connections in the peripheral nervous system and perhaps in all circuits involved in involuntary actions do not influence our state of happiness.

This relationship between the changes in the strength of connections and affect is partly the result of a circularity in definitions. Positive reinforcement is, of course, pleasant and according to the present theory always causes increases in connection strength, whereas negative reinforcement is unpleasant and is postulated to cause decreases in the strength of connections.

From the preceding paragraphs it might be inferred that changes in the strength of neural connections form the physiological basis for pleasure and happiness. It is very difficult, however, to imagine how such cellular events could reach consciousness. One could speculate about a humoral substance released whenever connections were being strengthened, that circulated throughout the brain and caused the firing of specific neurons that signaled happiness. So far no one has, however, found any indication for such "happy juice."

Another alternative is that the mean firing rate of neurons throughout the brain forms the physiological substrate for happiness, inasmuch as it usually is assumed that neuronal firing is the basis for all sensations. The firing rate is well correlated with the changes taking place in the strength of connections, as discussed in this chapter. The correlation breaks down only for neurons that have been resting for prolonged periods of time and consequently are no longer showing much increase in the strength of their connections, in contrast to neurons that have been resting for only a short time and are showing large increases. A problem with this possibility is the elicitation of responses related specifically to affect, such as smiling, frowning, crying, or even reporting verbally "I feel happy," when asked. How does information about the mean firing rate around the brain converge on the neurons responsible for triggering these responses? We could again postulate a converging network of neurons, as needed in the simple analysis at the beginning of the chapter, but coming from all neurons capable of influencing affect. As mentioned before, however, there is no evidence for such a network.

At present I have no solutions for this problem. The rest principle seems to account admirably for the more mechanical functions of the brain, including instrumental learning covered in this and the previous chapter. There are, of course, several solutions that would solve this problem, but rather than invoking astral bodies, homunculi, or even "happy juice" for the present theory I prefer to let the problem stand until there is more evidence available. It seems somewhat ironic that the rest principle fails to offer a plausible explanation for pleasure, because, as mentioned in the Foreword, this was the question that started me working on the rest principle in the first place.

As in Chapter 7, we might end by discussing the predictions that would be made from the use principle. The use principle does much better here than with drive- or stimulus-reduction learning and is able to account properly for stimulus-seeking behaviors. As mentioned previously, the rest principle is virtually the same as the use principle for rates of firing below r_{opt}, and consequently all the predictions from the rest principle for behaviors involving such low levels of stimulation would apply to the use principle. Both principles predict that firing infrequently used connections such as those at the top of sensory pyramids would be positively reinforcing. This also means that the use principle models for infrequently used neurons, such as the computer simulations by Kohonen, Lehtiö, and Rovamo (1974), and Kohonen et al. (1977) for the functioning of cortical units recording the memory of visual input (e.g. faces), would also work with the rest principle. The "additional assumption" also can be affixed to use principle theories, as has sometimes been done, and with it, these theories also would predict that sensory deprivation would weaken connections and subjects would leave experiments in which such deprivation was imposed.

For rates of firing above r_{opt}, however, the use principle again has problems. For this principle the curve relating the net change in the strength of connections to the rate of firing is a monotonically increasing function. There would therefore be no optimal level of stimulation for causing increases and similarly no optimal levels of change, complexity, novelty, or information flow. Connections also would become stronger the longer the duration of stimulation, regardless of intensity, although the increase would be greater for stronger stimuli. Stabilized retinal images would become more intense rather than fading. Eye movements would be learned that maintained stimulation on the same receptor. Tracking might be learned to the direct output of receptors, but motion of the stimulus per se would not be the factor eliciting tracking: Motion detectors would tend to excite eye movements in the direction opposite to tracking so as to increase the relative motion of the stimulus across the retina. With the observed physiology of the parietal neurons receiving input from the periphery of the retina, the fixation reflex would not occur, and there would be some tendency to move the fovea away from the stimulus so that maximal peripheral stimulation would occur.

Because the use principle has no provision for weakening connections other than "forgetting" if the additional assumption is allowed, it must postulate that extinction occurs because of learning to do something else. Inasmuch as the affect during extinction is clearly negative, whereas that during acquisition with, say, food reinforcement, is positive, the physiological basis for pleasure could not be any of the neural events occurring during both acquisition and extinction, such as the strengthening of connections or the firing rate of the neurons involved. Arousal has been implied to be the basis by some use principle theorists. Although it is true that arousal may influence affect, arousal alone cannot account for happiness or pleasure, inasmuch as happiness can easily occur with low arousal (happy-content, happy-satisfied) and with high arousal (happy-excited).

In this and the preceding chapters I have tried to account for learning with the rest principle without making any assumption about the organization of the central nervous system. This rule has been violated only with the assumptions of lateral inhibition, which the theory itself predicts, and with hierarchical pyramids and the provisional possibility of inhibitory connections between modalities. In general the brain has been treated as if it were a homogeneous box of neurons with initially random connections. The success of this analysis in accounting for learning may be attributed to the antiquity of the basic learning phenomena on an evolutionary scale. Even a very primitive organism with a largely undifferentiated nervous system would have been able to learn to obtain food and other psychologically needed substances for which it had receptor systems, to escape strong stimuli, and to approach moderate stimuli while leaving prolonged stimulation and thus remaining generally active, if it incorporated the rest principle. This ability to be beneficial even in the absence of specialized brain areas is an essential requirement for any general principle postulated for nervous function. A principle that was only beneficial once a creature had, for instance, developed a complex cerebral cortex would never have evolved to play a general role.

Nevertheless, there has been considerable opportunity since the time of such primitive creatures for specialized structures in the brain to have developed. These would not do away with the basic principle but rather augment it. In Chapter 9 we consider some of the specialized structures that now exist and how they might function in a rest principle brain.

9 Brain Structures and Neuronal Organizations

At present our knowledge of the function of various brain regions is analogous to the aversive situation, discussed in Chapter 8, of having overuse of the bottom neurons of a pyramid and little activity in the top neurons. An enormous amount of research is being done on the question. To review all the studies, for instance, on the ventromedial hypothalamic nucleus would fill a book the size of this one. This is only one of many hypothalamic nuclei, and the hypothalamus is only one small region in the brain.

On the other hand, there are very few uncontroversial "facts" concerning the function of any brain structure. As an example of the current poor state of our knowledge, in research on the control of alcohol drinking by rats, probably the strongest conclusion that can be reached is that neurons releasing norepinephrine are involved. This conclusion is based primarily on the fact that destruction of these neurons often has been found to affect alcohol drinking. In some studies it increased drinking, in others it decreased drinking; but so far there have been relatively few studies showing no change.

The paucity of facts is to a large extent due to the technological problems involved in studying the internal functioning of the brain and its parts. There is a story that R. J. Senter used to tell to students thinking of going into physiological psychology, which went something like this:

Two groups of Martians landed on Earth. One group was composed of behaviorists, the other of physiological psychologists. By chance, both groups ended up in bars with identical large jukeboxes and, being intrigued by the flashing lights and the music, both groups decided to study these "creatures." The behaviorists performed various experiments with their machine, including putting coins (which the fleeing humans had left behind) into the slot and pushing the buttons. They recorded all the results and, in a relatively short period of time, were able to predict with almost absolute certainty the behavior of the jukebox.

The physiological group went about their investigation somewhat differently. They opened the back of the jukebox and tried tracing the wires and then understanding the function of the various relays, capacitors, and so on. As electricity was used quite differently on Mars, they were not very successful, and after many years of diligent study they were still unable to make the jukebox play music.

The plight of the Martian physiological psychologists is actually far better than that which was faced by their counterparts on Earth at the time Senter told the story. The most commonly used technique at that time for studying the function of a part of the brain was to cut or burn it out and then see what behaviors were affected. This might be compared to studying the jukebox by smashing parts of it with a rather large hammer. The other common technique, stimulation of brain structures, as used then, might be compared to dropping into the jukebox a section of railroad track connected to a high-tension wire. The knife-cut technique that became popular shortly thereafter would be analogous to studying the jukebox with a machete rather than a hammer. Single-cell recordings are equivalent to sticking a voltmeter blindly into the jukebox, with practically zero probability of ever being able to hit the same wire twice, or at two different locations. Electroencephalographic (EEG) recordings are equivalent to studying the effects of the jukebox on the static heard on a radio.

Much of the modern work on brain organization has been stimulated by the discovery that three compounds, norepinephrine, dopamine, and serotonin, which were thought to be transmitter substances, could be made to fluoresce. This made it possible to locate in the brain the neurons manufacturing and releasing these compounds. Bundles of these neurons were found, with their cell bodies in the brainstem, moving forward through the hypothalamic area and projecting to various parts of the brain.

Certain chemicals were also discovered that destroyed these neurons. At first, relatively nonspecific procedures were used that, for instance, destroyed not only most of the norepinephrine cells but also most of the dopamine and some of the serotonin neurons. The techniques have since become more selective; it is now possible to destroy one type without doing too much damage to others and, with the proper placement, to destroy only neurons of one type within only one bundle. Other pharmacological techniques were discovered that blocked the receptors for these compounds or disrupted the production or storage of these compounds in the neurons.

Despite these improved techniques, the results have been somewhat disappointing. The problem comes partly from the fact that not all the neurons using a particular transmitter are concerned in the same way with producing an effect: For instance, it now seems likely that norepinephrine neurons in the dorsal bundle have a different role than do those in the ventral bundle. Another problem is that there are a multitude of compensatory mechanisms that are activated when neuronal function is altered. Consequently, one often cannot be sure if an observed result is caused by the experimental procedure or by the compensatory process produced to counteract it.

Another problem has arisen because of the discovery of these techniques. The emphasis upon these three compounds has produced a rather distorted view of the brain. The number of neurons containing norepinephrine, dopamine, and serotonin represents only a small percentage of the total number of neurons in the brain, but one could get the impression from the current literature that these are practically the only transmitters present. Actually there are several dozen compounds now suspected as transmitters or modulators. A modulator is a compound that acts primarily not to cause or prevent firing in the postsynaptic neuron but rather to influence its response to transmitters. As discussed later, it seems likely that at least in some synapses norepinephrine and dopamine act more like modulators than like transmitters.

Despite the problems, progress is being made. Techniques have been improved and we are currently obtaining relatively good data about the organization and function of many brain structures. Nevertheless, the evidence for most structures is still inadequate for evaluating the *rest principle*. My purpose in this chapter and in Chapter 10, therefore, is not so much evaluation as it is trying to paint a general picture of how the rest principle brain may be organized. Of necessity, this will involve a large amount of speculation based on a variety of grounds, including: (1) the types of structures and organizations that would be most beneficial to a rest principle organism; (2) the structures that might have developed most easily during evolution; (3) the current physiological evidence for what structures exist, how they are organized internally, how they interact with other structures, and how they function; (4) generalizations from the functioning observed in simpler structures as to what might occur in more complex ones; and (5) the current behavioral data concerning the roles of various structures.

The specialization of the nervous system could be considered as starting with the development of neurons themselves. I am tempted to include some speculations about how neurons might have developed from cells specialized in excreting sodium from a primitive organism, but as this has little bearing on the rest principle, I begin with the centralization of the nervous system at a time when neurons and muscles already existed. Imagine neurons with dendrites extending into an appendage of an organism. Initially the axons innervate various muscles. A strong external stimulus is applied to the end of the appendage, exciting the neurons. Those causing responses other than withdrawal of the appendage are weakened by continual use, but the neurons innervating the muscle causing withdrawal remove the stimulation from themselves, are allowed to rest after firing, and therefore develop stronger connections on the muscle.

The use of a single neuron for both sensory input and motor output offers little possibility for any modulating influences and no chance for such coordinated output as removing excitation from competing muscles. It also is dependent on plasticity in the neuromuscular junction rather than that at synapses between neurons. Therefore, it would be advantageous, first, to have a two-neuron reflex arc, which depends on synaptic plasticity and provides a locus for other inputs (see Fig. 9.1, part *b*). A three-neuron arc would offer the additional advantage of coordinated responses (Fig. 9.1, part *c*).

The single-neuron arc requires no centralization; the neuron could be located only in the tip of the appendage. If all connections already were genetically determined, there also would be little or no advantage to centralization of the synapses of two- or three-neuron reflex arcs. The synapses could, for instance, be located near the tip of the appendage, and the axons from neurons in other areas could grow out to them. If the number of inputs from other areas is greater than the number of neurons directly involved in the reflex, this would require more growth of axons than if the synapses were centralized (in the jukebox analogy, the total length of wire used in the construction of the machine would be greater); on the other hand, the time required to make a response would be less if the synapses were not centralized.

In an organism employing the rest principle, however, the connections do not need to be genetically determined, and centralization would be very advantageous because it would allow all possible useful connections to be developed. The neuron from the tip of the appendage, and all other input neurons, must be directed in some way to grow axons to the central ganglion, and it must be possible to make contact with the output neurons in the ganglion. After that, genetic control is not needed: A huge number of connections form randomly inside the ganglion and those allowed to rest after use become stronger. Because relaxation of opposing muscles helps in the withdrawal response, the neuron from the tip would develop indirect inhibitory connections that would remove excitation from the opposing muscles just as the excitatory connections onto the withdrawal muscle develop. Because of the centralization and the very short distances between all targets, the initial production of "incorrect" connections would not be particularly wasteful. There also is little biasing as to which connections will become stronger. For instance, the best response to stimulation to the head end of an organism might well involve a motor response at the tip of the tail. Without centralization and in the absence of specific genetic control, the connections producing this response would be very unlikely to be developed. With central representation, the neurons producing the tail response are nearly as close to the input neuron as those for motor response in the head itself, and therefore the needed connection could easily be made and then strengthened when experience showed that this tail response was beneficial.

As various other types of sensory input and a multitude of responses are evolved, there would be increasing benefits to further centralization within a

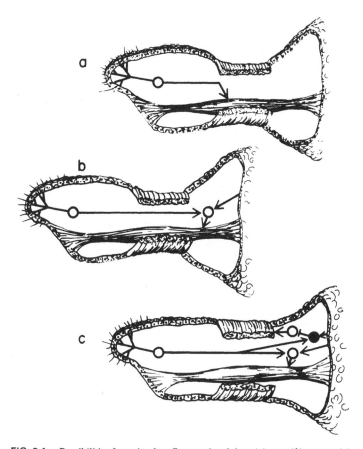

FIG. 9.1.   Possibilities for a simple reflex arc, involving: (a) one, (b) two, or (c) three neurons. The two-neuron arc offers the advantages of the plasticity of synapses and easier modulation by other inputs. The three-neuron arc going to the opposing extension muscles provides a coordinated response. The interposed inhibitory interneuron reverses the excitatory output of the receptor to inhibition of the input to these muscles. The rest principle would assure that the "correct" connections developed in all cases. As opposed to specific genetic specification, the rest principle control would benefit greatly from centralization of all synapses within a small area.

single ganglion. Because it is advantageous to have these sensory inputs at that end of a mobile animal that reaches new places first (i.e., at the head), the head ganglion would be favored as the location for this primary ganglion. Of course simple functions not requiring complex interactions would still be best controlled by peripheral ganglia closer to their input and output targets, thus reducing the transmission time along the neurons.

We now have an organism with a primary head ganglion or brain. This brain acts as a decision module functioning according to the rest principle and would allow the organism to display most of the basic behaviors mentioned thus far in this book, as discussed at the end of Chapter 8. All the modifications and additions augment this basic decision module but do not replace it.

The first modification to be discussed does not involve any changes in the basically random organization of the decision module but rather a modification of the blood system supplying part of the decision module and the addition (or development) of some cells that function as glands. For reasons that will become clear, this part of the brain might be termed the "leaky" region.

Hormonal output does not have to be controlled by the brain; many glands are capable of regulating their secretion without the direct involvement of neurons. Glands themselves can be sensitive to various substances and may vary output accordingly. There are distinct advantages for involving the brain in the regulation, however. The most obvious advantage of this centralization is the ease with which interactions with other stimuli and responses could be developed. Sensory input to the brain could then stimulate or suppress the output of hormones; conversely, hormone concentrations and the levels of other humoral substances also could influence behaviors directed by neurons in the brain. This was seen earlier in our S_h neurons, which were assumed to be influenced by humoral conditions related to hunger.

A second advantage is that negative-feedback control of hormone levels will develop automatically in a rest principle brain, provided only that some neurons have receptors for the hormone that influences their firing or are sensitive to other consequences of the hormone concentration and that the release of the hormone can be influenced in some way by neuronal output. This generally reduces the reliance upon specific control mechanisms and the genetic material needed to produce them.

As an example: Suppose that a gland releases a hormone that in turn stimulates a second gland to secrete some substance. This requires that a system be developed so that filling the receptors on the second gland with the hormone causes the second gland to increase its secretion. These receptors and the mechanism relating them to secretion could not be used by the first gland to regulate its output of the hormone, because they would produce a positive-feedback circuit: Output of hormone by the first gland would fill its own receptors, making it secrete more of the hormone, filling more of its receptors, and so on. Instead, a separate mechanism and perhaps a different type of receptor and second-messanger system would have to be developed for the hormone—a mechanism that inhibited secretion. Means would also have to be developed for assuring that the first gland had the inhibitory mechanism, whereas the second gland had the excitatory mechanism.

In contrast, if neurons are allowed to control the output of the first gland, negative-feedback control will develop regardless of whether the hormones increase or decrease the firing of the neurons. Initially there can be among the random facilitory and inhibitory connections of the neurons the makings for both negative- and positive-feedback circuits (i.e., those by which increased hormone levels lead to decreased hormone output and those by which they lead to increased output). Use of a positive-feedback circuit leads to additional more vigorous use, which according to the rest principle will weaken the connections involved. Use of a negative-feedback circuit removes its stimulus and therefore causes the strengthening of the connections in it. Thus, with a bit of experience, the hormone level automatically would be regulated in a negative-feedback manner.

This conclusion is a bit of an oversimplification and needs to be discussed further. First, I want to mention a simple way to determine whether a circuit involves negative or positive feedback, because this can become rather complicated, particularly with hormone control. Merely assign a value of $+1$ to all excitatory connections (e.g., when a substance causes an increased output of hormone) and a value of -1 to all inhibitory ones. If the product of these values is $+1$, the circuit acts as positive feedback; if the product is -1, the circuit acts as negative feedback. For instance, if a hormone excites ($+1$) a neuron to release a transmitter that inhibits (-1) the gland's secretion of the hormone, the product is $(+1) \times (-1) = -1$ and the circuit acts as negative feedback. As a more complex example, suppose hormone X excites ($+1$) neuron A; A inhibits (-1) neuron B; B inhibits (-1) neuroenodcrine cell C; C secretes a releasing factor that travels to the pituitary and stimulates ($+1$) the gland to release hormone Y; Y goes to a peripheral gland where it stimulates ($+1$) release of hormone X. The product is $(+1) \times (-1) \times (-1) \times (+1) \times (+1) = +1$, so the circuit acts as runaway positive feedback.

Now let us return to how the neuronal circuits would develop. The problem with the previous conclusion is that it neglects the interactions between the positive- and negative-feedback circuits. These have been investigated with computer simulations of the circuits shown in Fig. 9.2. Gland G secretes a hormone that indirectly stimulates neuron N_P in the positive-feedback circuit and

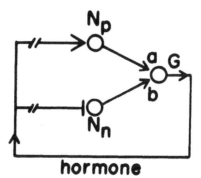

FIG. 9.2.   Circuitry modeled for controlling the hormone output of gland G via a positive-feedback path involving neuron N_p and a negative pathway including neuron N_n.

inhibits N_n in the negative-feedback circuit; both N_p and N_n then stimulate G via connections a and b. The strengths of these connections were made to obey the rest principle; the sensitivity of N_P and N_n also varied inversely with the preceding hormone level; and the output of G when the input to it was above threshold increased as a function of the duration of time since it last was activated. In a neuronal pool employing the rest principle, facilitory connections are likely to develop only from high threshold neurons seldom fired by the hormone to other high threshold neurons with an otherwise low rate of firing. Inhibitory connections develop best from neurons frequently (but not always) activated by the hormone onto spontaneously active neurons (or neurons with a high rate of firing due to other units). Therefore, N_P was given a positive threshold ($+10$ arbitrary units); N_n was given a negative threshold (-8) and thus fired whenever the inhibition times its sensitivity was reduced below this level.

Over a wide range of parameters, the following events occurred in the simulations. First, starting with equal strengths for connections a and b, the positive-feedback circuit was used repeatedly, causing an initial surge in the hormone level. Eventually connection a began weakening and the positive-feedback circuit began to stimulate G less frequently; the hormone level began falling, thus further reducing the ability of the positive-feedback circuit to excite G. Finally the hormone level and the sensitivity were reduced to the point that N_n fired and excited G. A certain hormone level was reached and never went far below this point. The strength of a remained close to the minumum needed to excite G, causing small surges in hormone whenever a happened to get a bit stronger. The strength of b in the negative-feedback circuit became progressively greater.

This dual regulation of hormone level, with both a strong negative-feedback circuit and a very weak positive-feedback circuit contributing, which the simulation suggested would probably develop with the rest principle, turned out to solve a problem inherent in negative-feedback circuits built with connections that themselves varied in strength according to negative feedback. An example of this problem can be seen in the regulation of glucose and insulin, a system that for the most part operates peripherally without central nervous system control. Basically, glucose stimulates secretion of insulin in the pancreas, which via insulin receptors on the cells throughout the body stimulates their uptake of glucose. This removes glucose from the blood, thus eliminating the stimulus to the gland to secrete insulin. The system therefore works in a negative-feedback manner. The number of insulin receptors, however, is also under negative-feedback control, such that continued high insulin levels reduce the number of receptors, whereas lack of insulin causes an increase in the number. In maturity-onset diabetes, and in various related animal models, the number of insulin receptors is greatly reduced, apparently as a result of previous prolonged high levels of insulin. The condition usually can be corrected by dietary controls that keep the insulin levels very low, thus causing the number of insulin receptors to increase again.

The problem amounts to maladaptive adaptation. A negative-feedback circuit with negative-feedback components will maintain the hormone level very precisely so long as no external factors interfere, but when some other factor causes the level to be too high or too low for long periods of time, the set point of the system shifts in the direction of the externally imposed level, because of the change in the components. Sometimes this may be advantageous. For instance, during a period when food is in short supply, the increase in the number of insulin receptors will increase the ability of the cells to capture and use glucose molecules that are in the blood. The adaptation of the set point would not, however, be advantageous for a system whose task is to maintain hormone levels within narrow limits.

It would be possible for other control processes to restore or maintain the set point of a nonneuronal system, but this control occurs automatically in a system using rest principle neurons, because of the dual regulation. As seen in the simulations, when the hormone level was externally kept at a very low point for a long period of time, connection a in the positive-feedback circuit was allowed to rest and become stronger. Consequently, when the system was again allowed to control the hormone level, the positive-feedback system was able to cause a surge in the hormone level (provided that the level sometime reached the threshold of N_P). The surge was proportional to the strengthening of a and caused a weakening of a to approximately the level it had before the period of externally imposed low hormone, and the hormone level was again maintained at its earlier level. The increase in the sensitivity of N_n to inhibition during the imposed low hormone period would have reduced the set point, but it was countered by an equal increase in the sensitivity of N_p to excitation, which kept the set point from being altered. The system also returned to its previous set-point after externally imposed high hormone levels. There were, however, limits to the system's ability to return (e.g., if the level was kept too low for too long, b eventually weakened from overuse and was unable to start the increase in hormone level thereafter).

There are, of course, a wide variety of circuits for regulating hormone levels that could develop with the rest principle. A different circuit would, for instance, be favored if the hormone receptors inhibited the firing of the neurons directly. The presence of lateral inhibition could also alter the circuit that would develop. Not all the systems that might develop with the rest principle avoid the adaptation problem, but unless extreme parameters are used, all those investigated managed to control the hormone level in a primarily negative-feedback fashion.

A final advantage of having the central nervous system regulate the level of a hormone is that it segregates the receptors monitoring the level from the gland secreting it. If the output of the gland were controlled by receptors to the hormone on the gland itself, or by neurons next to the gland, the concentration of hormone in the locality of the gland would be regulated, but not necessarily the concentration throughout the body. For instance, changes in the rate of blood circulation around the gland would vary the relationship between the local and general levels of the hormone. Placing the receptors on neurons in the brain and having the glands secrete into the venous blood from the brain, however, allows the general concentration in the body to be monitored, rather than the local concentration. On the other hand, there are suggestions that this segregation is not always maintained, in which case it could be used as a means for altering the hormonal response.

In addition to needing neurons whose firing is altered by hormonal concentrations, it is also necessary that the hormone reach the neurons. There is, however, a blood brain barrier that restricts the passage of many substances into the brain. For proper functioning of the hormone-regulating neurons, it would be necessary that the blood brain barrier be left out in the part of the brain where they are located. In fact there are a few small regions in the brain where there is no barrier and the permeability of the capillaries is similar to that found in nonneuronal tissues (Oldendorf, 1975). These regions are located near the neurons involved in the regulation of humoral substances.

No special neural architecture need be present for a negative-feedback control of hormones to develop. Therefore, the systems could be placed in the basic decision module. The brain area where they are located has to be leaky in two ways: Not only must the substance from the blood get into the area; the hormone produced must somehow get out. The secreting neuroendocrine cells must be able to release their hormone into the blood. Two systems have been developed. The magnocellular neuroendocrine cells that release vasopressin and oxytocin have axons extending into the posterior pituitary, where they secrete their hormones into the general blood circulation (see Hayward, 1977). The parvocellular neuroendocrine cells, which secrete various releasing and inhibiting factors, have axons terminating on the portal blood system that carries these factors to the anterior pituitary, where they influence the actions of the glandular cells.

In addition to controlling the level of hormones, an area of the brain with particularly free access to the blood would be ideally suited for controlling various other factors related to the blood. Thus we find that the hypothalamus, which is the area regulating hormones, also monitors the temperature of the blood and uses this information plus peripheral temperature signals to regulate the body temperature. Similarly, it monitors blood pressure in the brain and receives peripheral information about blood pressure to regulate the cardiovascular systems. Sexual behaviors are controlled here on the basis of monitored hormone levels and peripheral inputs such as genital stimulation. It monitors the glucose and fatty acid content of the blood; receives additional inputs such as those related to taste, smell, and stomach extension; and combines this information for use in the regulation of eating and the release of hormones in synchrony with it. Various inputs from the blood and periphery are used by the hypothalamus in its regulation of drinking. In summary, the hypothalamus is important for all activities in which one of the input factors comes from the blood and/or in which the response involves regulation of substances in the blood (see Hayward, 1977).

The importance of inputs from the blood often has been overemphasized, particularly in the case of consumatory behaviors. It is now clear that eating and drinking are not merely reflexes that are produced when the conditions in the blood indicate that more energy intake or more water is needed. Under normal conditions for humans and laboratory animals, the physiological controls from the blood play at most only a minor role. The hypothalamic glucose receptors can be blocked without interfering with normal eating; only in response to a day of starvation or to experimentally produced sharp reductions in blood glucose are the animals seen to be deficient (Woods & McKay, 1979). Infusing an animal with water causes only a rather small reduction in drinking (see Toates, 1979). Conversely, when an animal has a fistula implanted in its throat so that water or food that is consumed passes out of the body without reaching the stomach, the consumatory acts plus the stimulation produced by them are sufficient to terminate eating and drinking, though not so quickly as when the substances reach the stomach (Kraly, Carty, & Smith, 1978; Toates, 1979).

We have seen already how eating is controlled by a complex response chain; a similar response chain can be made for the control of drinking. There is, however, a second half of both these response chains that we have not yet considered: the mechanisms for *stopping* eating and drinking.

Sensory inputs related to stomach extension and also to the taste and/or feel of food and water enter the hypothalamus. According to the rest principle, neither alone will develop strong connections for stopping eating and drinking. Only AND gate neurons stimulated by the combination of stomach extension plus the taste/feel of food will develop inhibitory connections onto the neurons directing eating, whereas only AND gate neurons representing the combination of stomach extension plus the taste/feel of water will develop strong inhibitory connections onto the neurons directing drinking.

Let us consider the case with drinking. Remember that for a connection to become stronger it must be allowed to rest after use. This would not occur with connections from receptors signaling stomach extension. If the connections were facilitory and stimulated more drinking, their use would increase their own stimulus, thus producing a weakening. Even if the connections were inhibitory they would not be strengthened much. When the animal has had enough water to cause stomach extension, these receptors begin firing. Even if they manage to stop drinking by their inhibitory connections they do not remove the stomach extension. The stimulation remains; the connections continue being used and thus have little chance to grow.

The connections from the neurons representing the sensory stimulation from drinking onto the neurons eliciting drinking also would not grow. Facilitory connections, of course, are weakened because they increase their own stimulation. Inhibitory connections would not have much chance to develop, because they begin to fire when the animal is still very thirsty and is likely either to continue drinking despite the inhibition or to resume drinking immediately after the inhibition from the stimulation of the mouth and throat is gone. Therefore, the stimulation will continue, and the inhibitory connections will have little opportunity to rest and become stronger.

The AND gate neurons stimulated by the combination of stomach extension plus the taste/feel of water do not start firing when the animal first begins to drink because the stomach extension component is missing. Only after a considerable amount of water has been consumed are these neurons activated. Facilitory connections from them to the neurons eliciting drinking would be weakened because they increase their own stimulation. The inhibitory connections, however, would have a good chance of being able to rest after use. By the time they fire, the pathways eliciting drinking have already been weakened by prolonged use, and perhaps by some removal of the physiological factors related to thirst, inasmuch as some water already may have entered the circulation; in addition, competing responses that have been inhibited while drinking was taking place have grown stronger as a result of the enforced rest. Consequently, it is likely that when the AND gates begin to fire and momentarily inhibit drinking, the other responses will be strong enough to prevent the resumption of drinking after the inhibition from the AND gates is removed as the result of the taste/feel of water no longer being present. Because drinking is terminated, there is no further stimulation from the taste/feel of water and the AND gates are allowed to be silent; their inhibitory connections can rest and become stronger. Thus the AND gates for stomach extension plus the taste/feel of water become terminators for drinking. Similarly the AND gates for stomach extension, the taste/feel of food, and perhaps inputs from peripheral glucoreceptors develop strong inhibitory connections on the neurons eliciting eating.

With the development of such terminators and the growth of inhibitory connections from competing responses, the consummatory responses become progressively less dependent upon the physiological inputs related to the need for food and water. If the consummatory responses happen to be elicited, in the absence of hunger or thirst, by stimuli related to food or water or by spontaneous activity ("thoughts" of food and water or of eating and drinking), they still can get rest from the terminators and from inhibition from other responses.

Thus gradually the consummatory responses develop an autonomy. Although the physiological factors contribute after relatively long periods of deprivation, the factors usually eliciting the responses become the stimuli related to food and water, the absence of strong competing responses, and the current strength of the connections in the consummatory-response pathways determined by the *rest principle*. Here we see the rest principle in a new role: as the generator of long-term rhythms. When a meal or drinking bout has just ended, the strengths of the connections in the consummatory response pathways are reduced from having been used, so that it is very difficult to traverse them (but not impossible: e.g., the stimuli from the dessert may renew eating activity). During the periods after eating or drinking when the pathways are not being used, the connections become progressively stronger. It will be noted that some of the mechanisms for the rest principle, notably the change in the number of receptors, have a very long time course; the number of receptors continues growing over several days of disuse. As the connections grow with rest, it becomes progressively easier to elicit eating or drinking. After an hour or so, only exceptionally good-tasting food would trigger eating; after 3 or 4 hours, normal food will suffice and spontaneous activity may evoke looking for food; after much longer periods of deprivation, practically any food, even the most distasteful, will elicit eating.

It seems likely that the normal rhythms for eating and drinking are generated by this growth in response-pathway connections, coupled, in humans, with social factors that contribute stimuli related to food at the appropriate times for that society. If deprivation continues much longer than the normal separation between meals, the physiological factors will become progressively more important, up to a point. However, the pathways carrying the physiological information will themselves be weakened by continual use if the activity in them becomes too high. Consequently, there will be a maximum contribution from the physiological factors, and prolonging the deprivation will not increase this contribution further. There are reasons for believing that the factors in the blood contributing to the physiological input (e.g., glucose levels) also are limited and do not continue increasing beyond several hours of deprivation. The strength of the connections, however, is not limited nearly as soon and may not reach a maximum until several days of deprivation. Consequently, the strength of the connections would be responsible both for the additional increases in the response produced by very long deprivation and for the short-term increases, with the physiological factors being important only in the middle range. This is hard to verify with eating and drinking per se because of the detrimental effects of long-term deprivation of physiologically needed substances but is suggested by the research on the consumption of particular flavors.

To examine the consumption of such specifically flavored substances, let us look again at the consumatory response chains. They are controlled not by a single strand of neurons but rather by multiple parallel pathways with somewhat different inputs. This becomes increasingly pronounced as the responses develop autonomy. Once eating can be elicited by stimuli related to food, it may at one time, for instance, be produced by the stimuli related to pea soup; at the next meal it may be elicited by chicken; and so on. Each separate pathway will be strengthened with experience. The individual will have a pea soup consumption pathway and a chicken consumption pathway if extended experience has been obtained with these substances. Having been raised in America, I have a peanut butter consumption pathway, but most Finns do not, because peanut butter generally is not available in Finland. Incidentally, each food will develop its own terminator because the taste of the food was one factor contributing to the AND gates. Of course, these pathways for different foods do not remain completely separate; they all contribute to the general pathway, and they probably cluster together according to the similarity of the stimuli, so that all sweet substances have a common convergence pathway. Nevertheless, a fair amount of independence is maintained. As a result, it is possible to weaken selectively the consumatory pathway for a particular food. After having had pea soup for lunch, you are less likely to have "eating" elicited at dinner by pea soup again. The pea soup pathway has not had as much time to rest as, for instance, the chicken pathway and can only be fired after a longer period of total food deprivation when the general pathway has become stronger. After a few days of having only pea soup to eat, the very thought of it would "turn you off," and only very long periods of total food deprivation and strong input from the physiological components could induce you to eat another meal of pea soup. The same thing can happen for more general classes of foods: I understand that after a prolonged time on Weight Watchers' program, vegetables in general can become distasteful.

Conversely, deprivation of a particular type of food for which you have already developed a strong pathway can lead to increased desire for this food, a phenomena I have referred to previously as a "deprivation effect" (Sinclair & Senter, 1968). This is frequently mentioned by individuals who have left the region where they were brought up. A professor from New England, living in Oregon, complained of a "Maine lobster deprivation effect." I personally suffer from a severe "peanut butter deprivation effect."

Deprivation effects occur, according to the rest principle, because the pathways related to the specific substances grow progressively stronger as long as the substances are not present and the pathways are not used. My pea soup pathway gets used and thus temporarily suppressed nearly every Tuesday (due to the regularity of our food service at the laboratory), the chicken pathway every Friday, but the peanut butter pathway is almost never used and weakened. The long time course for these deprivation effects, apparently not reaching asymptote until after several weeks of deprivation, can only partially be accounted for by the long time course for the development of supersensitivity; and additional factor slowing their growth could be partial use of the specific pathways when foods with relatively similar stimulus properties are consumed. Eating salted peanuts may cause some firing in my peanut butter pathway and thus slow its development of supersensitivity.

Deprivation effects have been better documented for the drinking of flavored solutions. Rats (Sinclair & Senter, 1967; 1968) and monkeys (Sinclair, 1971) that are given free access to an alcohol solution as well as to water, and then deprived of alcohol, show a dramatic increase in their alcohol consumption when the alcohol is first returned. They begin drinking the alochol immediately (even though rats normally seldom drink during the day). Because of short-term factors, such as the terminator AND gates, animals do not finish weakening their alcohol consumption pathways back to normal during the first drinking bout or even during the first postdeprivation day; instead, their daily alcohol consumption returns only gradually to the predeprivation level during the first week to 10 days. The deprivation effect only grows slowly during the period without alcohol, again requiring more than a week to reach asymptote (Sinclair et al., 1973). This suggests that the connections in the pathway continue growing in strength for a similar period of time; the time course is relatively similar to the development of disuse supersensitivity. Because the effect apparently is caused by not using the alcohol pathway, it does not disappear again with prolonged deprivation, as would have been expected if it were caused, for instance, by alcohol withdrawal or by the firing of a pathway. Of course, it is necessary first to have the alcohol consumption pathway develop before deprivation can have any effect; consequently, the size of the deprivation effect increases as a function of how long the animals have had access to alcohol before it is taken away (Sinclair & Senter, 1968). Rats also develop deprivation effects for saccharin, quinine, citric acid, and salt solution (Wayner et al., 1972).

The development of deprivation effects, according to the rest principle, is not restricted to taste stimuli or to consumatory behaviors. Instead, it is a general property of any neural pathway. Use weakens connections in all pathways, and deprivation-induced rest will strengthen the connections again. Consequently, it would be predicted that for all responses, making the response causes a temporary weakening of the tendency to make it again, whereas prolonged inability to make it increases the response tendency. The experimental evidence suggests that this is true. Depriving animals of the opportunity to run in a wheel temporarily increases their subsequent wheel running (Premack, 1962). A similar effect is found with lever pressing (Premack & Bahwell, 1959). Rats kept in isolation show an increase in subsequent socializing with other rats. The increase in sexual activity caused by deprivation (e.g., Beach & Jordan, 1956) could be seen as another example. The weakening caused by use could account for spontaneous alteration in a T-maze: If a satiated rat is placed in a T-maze, allowed to wander into one of the arms, and then gently placed back in the "start" position, it will generally go into the opposite arm on the second trial (Dember & Fowler, 1958). The connections activated in going to the left on the first trial are weakened by use; consequently those involved in the opposite response, going to the right, are easier to traverse and more likely to be used on the second trial.

A common factor, rest principle control of the strength of connections, is thus involved in producing each of these compensatory behaviors and also in the deprivation effects for specific flavors and for food and water. Evidence that a common factor is involved can be seen in several similarities between these various behaviors, such as the time course for responding to return to normal, but the strongest evidences comes from the peculiar finding that one species, the golden hamster, fails to compensate for deprivation of alcohol (Sinclair & Sheaff, 1973), food (Silverman & Zucker, 1976), water, and saccharin (Sinclair & Bender, 1978) and also fails to show spontaneous alternation (Sinclair &

Bender, 1978). A possible explanation for why hamsters fail to show these compensatory behaviors is discussed in the section on the hippocampus. A relationship between the alcohol-deprivation effect and spontaneous alternation was also seen in rat strains developed for high and low preferences for alcohol (Sinclair, 1979). After deprivation, the AA's (those with a high preference) return to their normal level of consumption much more slowly and also show a reduced rate of spontaneous alternation; both results would be caused by their having less weakening of connections with use. Having the connections in the alcohol consumption pathway grow weaker at a slower rate when they are used but grow stronger at a normal rate during rest would also cause a higher general level of alcohol drinking.

These ideas take us a long way from the old switchboard model for behavior in which each stimulus was wired directly into its response and from the related view of homeostatic control in which the physiological inputs signaling hunger or thirst triggered eating or drinking as reflexes. External stimuli and internal ones such as those related to physiological needs still can, of course, bias which behaviors will be performed, but now a large degree of control is exercised by the current strength of the connections. This autonomous control is likely to predominate particularly in a relatively unchanging environment such as rats usually encounter in the laboratory.

I am afraid I have wandered rather far from the topic of specific brain areas. Most of my own research has centered on consumatory and compensatory behaviors, especially the alcohol-deprivation effect, and I become carried away when discussing it. Now let us return to brain regions, which are illustrated in Fig. 9.3.

As we have seen so far, a nonspecific organization of rest principle neurons handles most tasks very well. It has, however, one distinct failing: Connections are always susceptible to weakening by overuse. This "down-plasticity," which is very useful in removing a response that is no longer effective, also allows all the sensory processing and response programs to be destroyed. For instance, suppose that a primitive rest principle animal learned to swim toward the smell of a particular chemical when it was hungry. If once the animal happened to find the chemical-emitting food embedded in a hole where the animal could not reach it, the animal would be able to extinguish the response and thus eventually give up trying to get to this food. Unfortunately, the animal might also lose its ability to smell this chemical and to differentiate it from other smells, as well as the ability to go to other sources of the food emitting this chemical in the future, and even the ability to swim. The connections in the systems responsible for these functions would be overused and weakened while the animal was trying to get to the embedded food. Obviously, it would be advantageous to limit the down-plasticity in these systems and allow only the connections in the central decision module to be weakened.

Fortunately, the potential for weakening connections inherent in the rest principle can be circumvented easily. All that is needed is the presence of a large number of inhibitory interneurons for supplying some form of self-inhibition to the pathways. During the last few years there has been a "quiet revolution in our concepts of synaptic organization" (Schmitt, Dev, & Smith, 1976) that shows it is much easier than one would have supposed previously to supply self-inhibition to a pathway; it has shown also the extensive use of such inhibition in sensory input systems. The traditional view of neurons has been that they are excited and inhibited by synapses onto their dendrites and cell bodies; the postsynaptic electrical potential from these synapses summate at the beginning of the axon, determining whether or not an all-or-none action potential will be generated. If it is generated, it travels down the axon to the synaptic endings where it causes the release of transmitter. To use such neurons for supplying self-inhibition requires organizations such as those shown in Fig. 9.4 a and b, with a separate inhibitory neuron for each pathway neuron. It is now clear, however, that this is only one of many ways in which neurons can function. In the olfactory bulb, for instance, there are granule cells that have no axons (Shepherd, 1978); the amacrine cells in the retina also have no axons. Both act to produce self-inhibition (and lateral inhibition) on the pathway neurons through dendrodendritic synapses that involve only local graded electrical potentials rather than action potentials. The role of the granule cells in the olfactory bulb is shown in Fig. 9.4c. The presence of an odor excites receptor cells, which then excite mitral cells. In the figure, the dendrite of mitral cell M_1 has been excited. The electrical change in M_1 excites the dendritic spine of granule cell G, which then feeds back inhibition on M_1 and also inhibits other mitral cells such as M_2.

Lateral inhibition is beneficial regardless of whether neurons employ the rest principle. When there is input to one pathway, silencing of adjacent pathways increases the signal-to-noise ratio, and this aids in the reception of the signal by higher neurons. The importance of self-inhibition is apparent only with the rest principle; because continual repetitive use is suppressed, the connections along the information-carrying pathway cannot be greatly weakened by the prolonged presence of a strong stimulus. Furthermore, the inhibition produced by the granule cells is long-lasting relative to the excitation impulse, thus providing time for the recovery of strength.

Also in the olfactory bulb, where the receptor cell synapses onto the mitral cell, is another type of interneuron, the periglomerular cell, that forms the type of junction shown in Fig. 9.4d. When the receptor cell excites the mitral cell, it also excites the periglomerular cell, which then inhibits the mitral cell and may contribute lateral inhibition to other mitral cells. At least some of the periglomerular cells release dopamine (Halász, Hökfelt, Ljungdahl, Johansson, & Goldstein, 1977), in contrast to the olfactory granule cells that probably release GABA (Shepherd, 1978). A relatively similar arrangement of interneurons (hori-

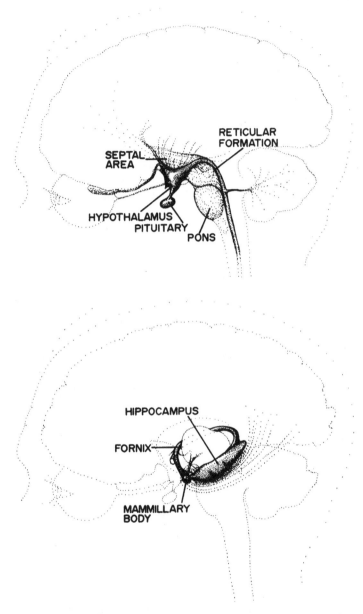

FIG. 9.3. The basic regions of the human brain. Each frame emphasizes a different set of regions, roughly representing the types of organizations discussed in this chapter. Upper left: the most primitive parts of the brain, probably including much of the basic decision module. Upper right: the somewhat newer areas that develop around and above the oldest parts; many of these newer areas contain profuse lateral inhibition that should restrict weakening with overuse. Lower left: the hippocampus and some related structures. Lower right: the newest portions of the brain.

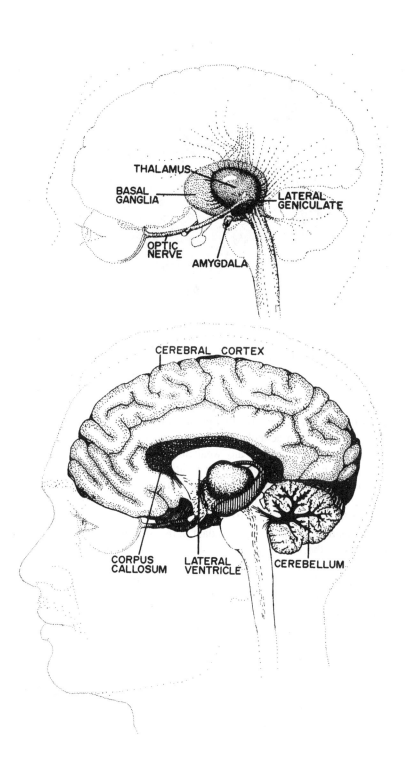

THALAMUS

BASAL
GANGLIA

LATERAL
GENICULATE

OPTIC
NERVE

AMYGDALA

CEREBRAL CORTEX

CORPUS
CALLOSUM

LATERAL
VENTRICLE

CEREBELLUM

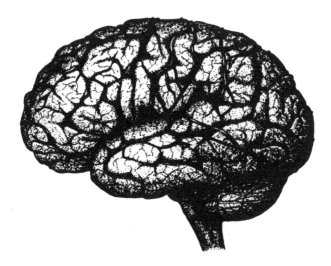

FIG. 9.3. (*Continued*) An external view of the brain.

zontal and amacrine cells) is found in the retina, and again there is a population of dopamine-releasing interneurons (Ehinger, 1977; Iuvone, Galli, Garrison-Gund, & Neff, 1979). The actions of dopamine at these junctions remains to be determined, but in analogy with its actions in ganglia (Kobayashi et al., 1978; Libet, 1977) it is possible that dopamine first prevents weakening by overuse (by an inhibitory action) and then actually makes the junction easier to fire for a while thereafter. This could counteract any weakening that still occurred at other synapses and might be partially responsible for positive afterimages in the visual system. It would also predict positive aftereffects in the olfactory system, for which I know of no evidence. A general discussion of the possible role of dopamine neurons follows in Chapter 10.

Inhibitory interneurons are also very abundant in the thalamic relay nuclei for sensory input, such as the lateral geniculate nucleus in the visual system (see Singer, 1977). The relays do little to alter the characteristics of the information, but again the lateral inhibition serves to increase the signal-to-noise ratio. Anatomical evidence suggests the presence of symmetrical dendrodendritic synapses between the pathway neurons and the inhibitory Golgi type II interneurons, similar to those between the mitral and granule cells (Fig. 9.4c), and also arrangements similar to that involving the periglomerular cells (Fig. 9.4d). Although the functional correlate of these synapses has not yet been identified, the usefulness of such self-inhibition on the sensory pathways in preventing their weakening from overuse is predicted by the rest principle. As discussed in Chapter 10, the various inhibitory interneurons in the thalamic relay nuclei appear to play a critical role in attention and arousal.

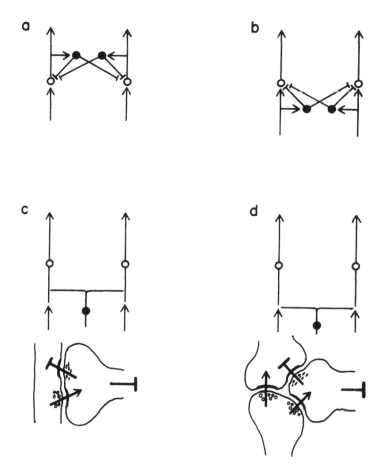

FIG. 9.4. Organizations providing inhibition with conventional axodendritic synapses (a and b) and dendrodendritic synapses (c and d). Recurrent self-inhibition and lateral inhibition of the type provided by basket cells in the hippocampus is shown in a. Feed-forward inhibition is shown in b. In c, activation of the dendrite of the (vertical) pathway neuron excites a dendrite of the (horizontal) inhibitory interneuron, which supplies self-inhibition to the dendrite exciting it, via the reciprocal synapse (shown in detail below) and lateral inhibition to other pathway neurons. In d, the input axon excites both the pathway neuron and the inhibitory interneuron, in the glomerulus arrangement shown in detail below. The inhibitory interneuron then inhibits the pathway neuron and supplies lateral inhibition to other pathway neurons. The lateral inhibitory components increase the signal-to-noise ratio. The purpose of the self-inhibitory components is clear from the rest principle: They protect the pathways by retarding weakening from overuse and may in some circumstances allow a subsequent net increase in the strength of synapses that have been used.

Inhibitory interneurons also are present in the motor output systems. For instance, the Renshaw cells in the spinal column provide recurrent inhibition, including a self-inhibition component of the type shown in Fig. 9.4a to the motoneurons (Eccles, 1967; Granit & Rutledge, 1960). Incidentally, although there is not enough evidence for concluding exactly how the rhythmic output needed for locomotion is generated, some of the models currently under consideration are dependent on the strength of neural connections being controlled by the rest principle to the extent that they become weaker during use and regain their strength while inhibited and resting (Grillner, 1975; Pearson, 1976).

In addition to protecting the sensory input and motor output pathways from weakening, it also would be advantageous to protect the central sensory analyzing and motor program systems with inhibitory interneurons. Such interneurons also would serve another purpose: providing a sort of internal local reinforcement for the formation of associations. Most of the associations we have considered so far have been strengthened as a result of external contingencies. For instance, the association of stimuli related to hunger and those related to food in the S_{h+food} AND gate neuron was strengthened because only this combination of stimuli was consistently present when eating would remove the stimulation. Similarly, the AND gate for stomach extension plus the taste/feel of water would develop because it could remove its own stimulation, via inhibitory connections to the neurons eliciting drinking.

It would be advantageous to be able to form associations between stimuli that tended to occur together even when such external contingencies do not exist. A simple example of how this could be done is shown in Fig. 9.5. Assume that the threshold for P is initially high enough that input from two G cells is needed to fire it. If, for instance, G_a and G_c occur simultaneously, they will be able to excite P. P then excites the inhibitory interneuron B, which then inhibits P and the G cells. As a result of this inhibition the connections from G_a and G_c onto P, and to a lesser extent the connections onto G_a and G_c, would become

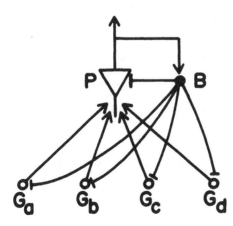

FIG. 9.5.   A simple organization for the formation of associations.

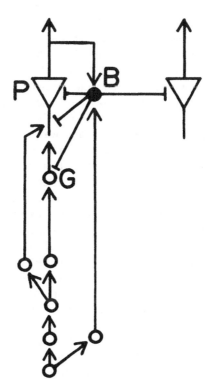

FIG. 9.6.   Probable neuronal organization related to the CA3 pyramidal cells (*P*) of the hippocampus. *B* = basket cell; *G* = granule cell. For simplicity the multiple inputs to *P* from different granule cells and the multiple afferent inputs to *B* and *G* are not shown. Compiled from Andersen, 1975; Andersen et al., 1963; Andersen, Gross, Lømo, and Sveen, 1969; Eccles, 1967; Lopes da Silva & Arnolds, 1978; Spencer & Kandel, 1968.

stronger. If G_b is fired at times when none of the other G cells is active, it will be able to go on firing indefinitely without exciting P and without receiving any inhibition from B; therefore, its connections will grow weaker. P eventually will become an AND/OR gate, firing whenever G_a, G_c, or both are present.

Although it now seems likely that organizations similar to that shown in Fig. 9.5 occur in other places within the brain such as the neocortex, it was first identified in the hippocampus (Andersen, Eccles, & Loyning, 1963; Eccles, 1967; Lopes da Silva & Arnolds, 1978). P represents the large pyramidal cells, B is a basket cell probably releasing GABA (Roberts, 1974), and the G units are the granule cells. (The granule cells in the hippocampus, which are excitatory, should not be confused with the granule cells in the olfactory bulb, discussed earlier, which were inhibitory). The actual organization of the neurons in the hippocampus is somewhat more complicated than that shown in Fig. 9.5: A summary of the most likely connections is shown in Fig. 9.6.

That the hippocampus reacts to stimuli being associated (e.g., by classical conditioning) has been demonstrated (Berger, Alger, & Thompson, 1976; Segal & Olds, 1973). For instance, pyramidal and granule cells that did not respond to either a tone or an air puff to the cornea did respond to the pairing of the two stimuli and subsequently to the tone alone. Incidentally, it would be predicted that, unlike the development of CRs, the firing of the hippocampal units would occur best if the stimuli were presented simultaneously.

The neuronal organization shown in Fig. 9.6 also would produce expectations (e.g., event C is expected to follow event B) on the basis of experience (B usually being followed by C) and would evaluate whether the expectations are met. In Chapter 5 it is shown how topological mapping would develop in a system with lateral inhibition because spatially adjacent stimuli are likely to be experienced one after another. In the same way, it is likely that events that occur sequentially will come to elicit firing in adjacent hippocampal pyramidal cells because of the existing lateral inhibition through the basket cells. Suppose that event B is always followed by event C. Event C already elicits firing in P_C, which has (via its basket cell) strong lateral inhibitory connections on P_B and on other adjacent pyramidal cells but not on the distant cell P_N. Event B can elicit firing in both P_B and P_N (via granule cell G_B). Its firing of P_B is followed by inhibition from both the basket cell of P_B and the basket cell of P_C, because P_C is fired immediately after event B. Because the lateral inhibition from P_C does not reach to the distant P_N, there is only one source of inhibition when B fires P_N (i.e., the basket cell from P_N). Therefore, the connection G_B–P_B will be strengthened more than G_B–P_N, because more inhibition is imposed on P_B (see Fig. 9.7).

Over the course of having event C follow B repeatedly, the lateral inhibitory connection from the basket cell B_B excited by P_B to P_C will become progressively stronger, because whenever B_B fires its source of excitation, P_B is inhibited first by the output of B_B itself and then by the firing of B_C that follows. The growth of B_B–P_C causes an initial inhibition to P_C before C can cause it to fire. This suppression of P_C after event B amounts to an expectation that event C will follow B. As long as expectations are met, the output of the system is reduced. If, however, event X follows B, there will be a high amount of output from the system from P_X. First, there is no inhibition from B_B onto P_X to retard its firing, and second, the event that normally preceded X did not occur to inhibit P_X.

It is also possible that the feed-forward inhibition from afferents onto the basket cells shown in Fig. 9.6 could contribute to the suppression of P_C (i.e., to the expectation). Suppose that there are two types of basket cells: the recurrent ones stimulated by the pyramidal cells and the feed-forward ones stimulated by the afferents; also suppose that the former inhibit the latter. Any afferent stimulated by event B will develop strong excitatory connections onto the feed-forward basket cell inhibiting P_C, because it is inhibited after use. Event B excites the connection; event C excites P_C, which excites its recurrent basket cell, which then inhibits the feed-forward basket cell.

With both mechanisms, the expectation could extend beyond just the next event: B might cause some inhibition also to P_D, P_E, and so on, although not so much as to P_C. The inhibition to all the pyramidal cells representing expected

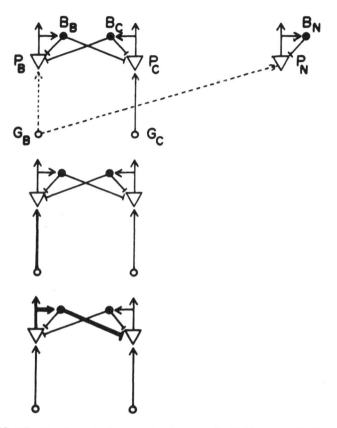

FIG. 9.7. Development of an expection that event C will follow event B. First, sequential events, B and C, are more likely to excite adjacent pyramidal cells: $G_B\text{-}P_B$ grows more than $G_B\text{-}P_N$ because of the inhibition from B_C on adjacent P_B but not on the distant P_N. Second, the inhibitory connection from B_B to P_C grows because of the double inhibition of P_B, first from B_B and then from B_C when event C follows event B. The expectation is seen as a suppression of the firing of P_C if B precedes C.

events could remove inhibition from them onto pyramidal cells representing unexpected events, which otherwise might have been caused by spontaneous activity. Consequently, an unexpected event could produce more firing if it occurred in the course of a well-learned series of events than if it occurred in isolation.

The firing of pyramidal cells should be partly determined, according to these analyses, by learned expectations, such that expected stimuli will produce little output, whereas novel or unexpected events will cause more firing, as found to be true (Vinogradova, 1975). During the course of an experiment in which there is a reliable sequence of events, the pyramidal cells initially should show a high output because no expectations are present; subsequently, as the expectations develop, the firing should subside. If the sequence is altered, the output would again increase, probably to a higher level than was found at the beginning of the experiment. This may help to explain the role of the hippocampus in extinction. In general, it has been found that lesioning of the hippocampus does not hurt the acquisition of simple discrimination tasks (in line with the previous discussion on the lack of effect of expectations per se on choosing the proper response [p. 116]). Hippocampal lesions do, however, increase the resistance to extinction (see Kimble, 1975). The output from the hippocampus is excitatory and goes to the lateral septal area, the brainstem and other parts of the "decision module" (Lopes da Silva & Arnolds, 1978). The increased excitation here will raise the rate of reverberation and may contribute to the behavioral excitation seen with frustration when expectations are not met. This in turn will increase the rate at which S-R connections in the decision module are weakened and thus facilitate extinction. Suppose that an animal has learned to expect food when it bar presses. During extinction, when the response does not produce food, the connections involved may be weakened by the continuing presence of the same stimuli and the subsequent bar presses. Diffuse excitation of the system as a result of hippocampal output could increase reverberation within the circuits; this will increase the overuse of the connections involved in triggering bar pressing and hasten their weakening. If the external contingencies had not really changed and the failure to obtain food was caused, for instance, by the animal's not pressing hard enough, the hippocampal output again would be beneficial, because the animal would try the response with greater vigor, thus pressing harder and obtaining food. Removal of the hippocampus should therefore lessen frustration-induced excitation and delay extinction. It also would reduce the rate of spontaneous alternation, inasmuch as reverberation supported by hippocampal output in the novel T-maze would be a major factor weakening the connections involved in the response chosen on the first trial. It is also possible that the greater excitation from the hippocampus when the rat faces the novel arm of the T-maze on the second trial might help to activate entering this arm and contribute to alternation.

It should be cautioned that these speculations do not model the modern hippocampus, nor are they intended to do so. All details concerning the broad-scale organization of the hippocampus, such as the differences between the CA3 and CA1 regions, have been omitted. Even the relatively complicated neuronal organization shown in Fig. 9.6 is probably much simpler than the real organization. The output of the hippocampus has been treated in a deliberately vague manner (e.g., its possible innervation of inhibitory interneurons in some septal regions [McLennan & Miller, 1974] has not been considered). It seems likely that one of the major functions of the modern hippocampus is to serve as one of the interfaces between the neocortex and the lower brain areas. This aspect has been omitted because I wished to consider how a primitive hippocampus might have functioned before the development of the neocortex.

My major purpose has been to show how a system for storing associations and expectation might be made rather simply from rest principle components, and how such a system could have benefited a primitive organism, augmenting the capabilities of the basic decision module. The relationships to the modern hippocampus are, I think, nevertheless interesting and suggest that these functions may still be in its repertoire today.

The decision module is ill-suited for storing associations and expectations. Random facilitory innervation cannot form associations or expectations without external contingencies, and those that do form are susceptible to destruction if the contingencies are changed for a while. Scattering inhibitory neurons randomly among the facilitory ones allows associations and expectations to form wherever a pathway has been used enough to develop an inhibitory surround, as seen with classical conditioning; they can form, however, only with components of the pathway itself.

In order to store associations and expectations on a continual systematic basis requires a deviation from merely random neuronal organization. It is necessary to have large neurons with extended dendritic trees available for receiving inputs from huge numbers of afferents; the large neurons must be located near one another and probably need to be arranged in some orderly geometric pattern (for instance, spread out on a surface); and there must be ample inhibitory interneurons near the large neurons. The innervation of the interneurons and their innervation of the large neurons will occur automatically with the rest principle, as seen in Chapter 5, provided that at some stage in development the large neurons are relatively active. Once the inhibitory connections have been formed, the pyramidal-basket cell complexes are ready to store associations from among the afferent inputs reaching them, supplying reinforcement in the form of inhibition to whatever afferents can turn them on and developing expectations primarily because of the geometrical arrangements of the pyramidal cells. The development of a primitive hippocampus does require, therefore, more genetic specification than the decision module did, but the requirements are still quite modest.

The consequences, however, are not at all modest. The ability to form the hippocampus-type of neuronal organization opens the door for dramatic new developments, culminating in the human cerebral cortex.

The ability to store associations may have seemed rather unimportant when I discussed it earlier; actually, it is very important. Such associations form the basis for all but the simplest sensory perception. Perhaps you have noticed that the stimuli used as examples when discussing the decision module per se generally have been very simple: a bell ringing, hunger, a light turning on, general stimuli related to food, and so on. The reason for this limitation is that such stimuli are the only ones that the decision module can react to selectively. It probably could not distinguish between an apple and a red flower, and it certainly would not have a general concept of "apple" that could be activated by red, green, or yellow apples. Such abilities require the formation of associations with a hippocampal type of neuronal organization.

Consider the matrix shown in Fig. 9.8 illustrating the topological map in the cortex of the retina. Each number represents a thalamic cell fired by light on the corresponding retinal field. Now imagine that these cells play the role of the afferent inputs in our model of the hippocampus and randomly innervate pyramidal cells with recurrent lateral and self-inhibition. Of all the pyramidal cells within a given region, P_A happens to receive the strongest inputs from 3, 8, 13, 18, and 23. If a vertical line is projected onto these fields in the retina, simple cortical cells 3, 8, 13, 18, and 23 all will fire; P_A will be activated and then its inhibitory neuron, I_A. I_A inhibits P_A, strengthening these inputs that managed to fire it and also inhibiting other pyramidal cells, thus preventing most of them from firing in response to this stimulus. Many of the rest principle models would state that the connections to these inhibited pyramidal cells would be weakened, because transmitter is being released and the receptors filled but the postsynaptic neuron is not fired. Because the inhibition from I_A prevents them from firing to this vertical line, even if their strongest inputs were also from 3, 8, 13, 18, and 24, they will have to settle for being activated by stimuli with slightly weaker connections on them. P_X, for instance, may be the first fired by 11, 12, 13, 14, and 15 (i.e., a horizontal line in these fields). This stimulus, incidentally, contains one of the components in the stimulus activating P_A, cell 13. Because P_X fired first to the horizontal line, then P_A, which is inhibited by I_X, has little chance of responding. The firing of cell 13 onto P_A without being able to fire P_A may cause some weakening of its connection. Vertical lines occur often enough

1	2	3	4	5
6	7	8	9	10
11	12	13	14	15
16	17	18	19	20
21	22	23	24	25

FIG. 9.8.   Matrix illustrating the afferent input to the visual cortex. Each number represents an afferent and also a corresponding retinal field. Afferents 3, 8, 13, 18, and 23, for instance, would oe activated by a vertical straight line.

in the real world for this weakening to be of little consequence; there are ample opportunities for 13 to participate in firing P_A and then having its connection strengthened by the inhibition from I_A. Suppose, however, that when P_A was first fired, there was also a spot of light exciting input 11, and thus 11 was able to contribute to the initial activation of P_A. Its connection with P_A also would have been strengthened. Like 13, its connection on P_A might be weakened when the horizontal line appeared, but unlike 13, 11 is seldom stimulated at the same time as 3, 8, 13, 18, and 23: Vertical lines with dots to the left are rare stimuli. Consequently, 11 may gradually lose its connection on P_A, and P_A would become a pure vertical line detector. Even if weakening does not occur when an input fails to activate a pyramidal cell, there will be a divergence caused by the frequent strengthening of connections related to straight lines: P_A still will become essentially a vertical line detector and P_X a horizontal line detector.

Which pyramidal cells become selectively activated by which lines will not be random. Instead, pyramidal cells fired by lines with the same orientation but differing retinal locations should be clustered together. The reason for this is the same as for topological mapping and depends on the external contingency that the stimulus most likely to follow a line with a certain orientation at one retinal location is a line with the same orientation at a different location or, more precisely, the same external line stimulus shifted to a new retinal position by eye movements or its own movement. Suppose a vertical line other than that already exciting P_A is presented and activates two pyramidal cells: P_B, which receives inhibition from I_A, and P_Y, which is out of the range of I_A. This line is then shifted to the position stimulating P_A. Both P_B and P_Y already will have received some inhibition from their own recurrent inhibitors, but P_B also will receive additional inhibition from I_A. Thus P_B is the more likely of the two to become a vertical line detector like P_A. Once P_B is partially established in this role, P_C, which receives inhibition from I_A and I_B, is very likely to become a vertical line detector as well, and I_C will help to strengthen the connections selectively activating P_A and P_B to vertical stimuli, Thus a chain reaction occurs so that eventually all pyramidal cells within the cluster with P_A will be vertical line detectors. A possible additional factor that could contribute to this development is rebound firing after release from inhibition, which would make a neuron in this cluster likely to fire when the others cease firing and inhibiting it. Inasmuch as this probably would occur when the vertical line moves to a retinal location out of the range of all the other units in the cluster, the neuron is likely to become selectively activated by this stimulus even if the afferents to it excited by this stimulus are not initially strong enough themselves to cause the neuron to fire.

These conclusions are in close agreement with the observed organization and function of the visual cortex (Hubel & Wiesel, 1959; 1962; 1963a; 1963b; 1965). The simple cortical neurons in the striate cortex that receive the output of the lateral geniculate nucleus in the thalamus do act as line detectors. The cortex is organized into columns perpendicular to its surface. The neurons within a column have profuse connections with one another but few connections with neurons in other columns. This columnar arrangement is ideally suited for the development of the clusters I discussed. In agreement with the conclusions, it has been found that the simple cortical cells within one column all respond to lines with the same orientation but with different retinal locations.

There is an apparent inconsistency in the experimental results as to the origin of line detectors. Because kittens with no visual experience show nearly the same arrangement of line detectors, it seemed likely that the development of the required selective innervation was innately controlled (Hubel & Wiesel, 1963a; 1965). Various sorts of experience, however, cause changes in the stimuli that can excite the cortical cells, suggesting that the pattern of innervation was not determined by genetics (Shinkman & Bruce, 1977). Most of the studies involved visual deprivation of some kind, and it was felt that perhaps the initial innervation was innate but that deprivation might destroy some connections. Spinelli and Jensen (1979) have now shown, however, that experience not involving deprivation alters the innervation. They trained kittens for 8 minutes daily on a visually signaled avoidance task with shock to the forearm. The rest of the time the kittens had normal visual experience. Nevertheless, dramatic changes were found in both the somatosensory and visual cortices, clearly reflecting the avoidance training. These changes involved responsiveness to vertical and horizontal lines, which had been used as the discriminative stimuli.

These results show that the selective innervation can be controlled by experience and thus are in general agreement with the proposal made here that the rest principle could account for the development of line detectors. There are two ways to reconcile this conclusion with the results suggesting innate determination of the connections. It could be assumed that there is a genetic program directing the growth of neuronal fibers and connections responsible for producing line detectors and that through a different process, possibly involving the rest principle, experience is able to change the connections, destroying some line detectors and forming others. A more parsimonious possibility is that experience before the eyes open is responsible for the "innate" innervation and therefore that only one process is involved. The process described here would require that lines of retinal cells be fired simultaneously, even before the eyes open and the external world provides line stimuli to cause such firing.

I would like to make a tentative suggestion for a way in which such firing patterns could be produced. While examining the hypothetical behavior of rest principle neurons lying in a plane with lateral inhibition, I realized that in the complete absence of patterned input the activity would be likely to become organized into waves of firing, radiating as concentric circles from some more or less accidental focus. Basically, the waves are generated because a firing neuron inhibits its neighbors and thus removes inhibition from itself, favoring its own continued firing and the silence of its neighbors; during the firing it becomes weaker by continued use and the neighbors become stronger because of inhibition-induced rest; a phase inversion eventually occurs so that the neighbors fire, whereas the original neuron and also a ring of neurons outside the neighbors are inhibited. With each new phase inversion the rings of firing and inhibited neurons move outward. Even on a flat plane the concentric rings would create nearly straight lines of simultaneous firing at large distances from the focus. On the spherical surface of the retina, the nonlinearity disappears more rapidly: At 90° from the focus, the concentric waves excite the same receptors as an external straight line projected onto the retina.

Originally I had thought this might be related to EEG activity, but the requirement that all units receive the identical external input (or no input), plus physiological evidence as to how EEG activity is generated, makes this unlikely, although it might still play a role in the waves from isolated cortical slabs. If, however, such waves did occur on the retina prior to eye opening, they could provide the "experiential" basis for the development of line detectors. In addition, unlike visual experience, there would be no more input from vertical and horizontal lines than from all other lines, in accordance with the initial lack of biasing for these orientations.

How the initial innervation of the visual system occurs is still unresolved. Nevertheless, the rest principle provides a means for development of line detectors without genetic specification and for the later development of new line detectors and higher feature analyzers with experience. Having specific detectors is, however, only half of the problem in perception. In addition there must be a process for generalizing from specific features. In the case of the line detectors, this is represented by the transformation from simple cortical cells that respond to lines with a given orientation at specific retinal locations to complex cells that respond to lines of this orientation regardless of their location. The major factor contributing to the development of the required innervation appears to be anatomical. The complex cells for a given orientation occur within a column of simple cells with the same orientation responsivity; the selective innervation occurs, therefore, because connections develop primarily between neurons within the same column. Nevertheless, a process similar to that modeled for the development of line detectors, but involving primarily temporal summation rather than spatial summation, also could contribute to the strengthening of the required connections. Because lines with the same orientation but different locations are most likely to follow one another as stimuli, the connections from simple line detectors with the same orientation are most likely to activate a complex cell that initially required the temporal summation of several inputs to fire it. With the strengthening of connections, such an AND gate neuron then would be transferred into an AND/OR gate neuron capable of firing to any of the separate inputs. The sequential activation of several simple cells (e.g., by a line moving across the retina) would still be expected to produce a greater response, as is indeed the case (Hubel & Wiesel, 1965). On the other hand, because of the proposed inhibitory connections between simple cells, a stimulus consisting of two parallel lines would not be expected to be generally more effective than a single line, as also was found.

These two processes, selective activation and then generalization, are repeated in similar fashion at higher areas of the visual cortex (Hubel & Wiesel, 1965). The effective stimuli become progressively more exact in terms of features (lines of a given orientation and length, right angles, angles with a certain movement, and so on) with "hypercomplex" and "higher-order hypercomplex" neurons, but more general so that various stimuli with the proper characteristics can fire the neurons.

The natural extension of these results leads to the development of specific feature analyzers and general "concept" neurons (e.g., "apple" analyzers and neurons that fire to all apples). There have been objections to this extension in the past (e.g., Feeney, Pittman, & Wagner, 1974), and attempts have been made to explain the functioning of the cortex in ways that do not involve the localization within separate neurons of the ability to recognize such specific stimuli (e.g., imagining that the cortex works like a hologram). The evidence in favor of specific feature analyzers has, however, been accumulating (see Buser, 1976). I have mentioned previously the cells in the visual system responding only to hands or to syringes of the right color when hungry. Units also have been found in the auditory cortex of squirrel monkeys and macaques that respond specifically to vocalization features of their own species.

Evidence in favor of the hierarchical sensory pyramids (as discussed in Chapter 8) needed for producing such feature analyzers has also been growing. One new method contributing to this evidence is the analysis of glucose uptake and thus neuronal activity, using positron-emitting isotopes (Fox, 1978). With this method he has shown that "Every step in the visual pathway does something new. Each step depends on the previous step." Four stations have been identified projecting from the visual cortex, down the temporal lobe, and eventually into the amygdala below the cortex. The first processes for characteristics such as shape, color, and size; the second integrates these into a whole; the third recognizes objects that have been seen before; and finally the amygdala relates objects with feelings. As Livingston pointed out (1967): "Feelings provide the 'go/no go' switch for all behaviors." Thus the amygdala acts as an interface between the neocortex and what I call the decision module. As mentioned before, other structures such as the hippocampus also seem to serve this function.

In summary, the genetically determined ability to develop the basic hippocampal type of neuronal organization allows associations to be stored systematically. This allows the development of feature analyzers. The genetically determined columnar arrangement facilitates generalization with "concept" neurons. The perceptual abilities thus produced provide the decision module with a better basis upon which to make decisions.

The advantages gained in providing the decision module with a neocortex seem somewhat analogous to those gained when a human is given a computer. Both the cortex and the computer are superior at storing large quantities of information on a relatively permanent basis, analyzing the information down to manageable and meaningful data and operating with little interference from emotions or physiological needs. The proliferation of the cortex seen in evolution has some parallels to the proliferation of computers in our modern world. Both the cortex and the computers function better the larger they are because the amount of information they can store is a function of size. In contrast, the decision module is limited in its capacity to store information not by size so much as by the fact that connections in it can easily be weakened.

All the perceptual advances are proposed to be based upon the ability of the hippocampal type of neuronal organization to form associations. It seems likely that the cortex has also capitalized on the second ability: to store expectations. Expectations amount to a crude sort of memory for temporal sequences of events. How this ability has been transformed into our capacity for laying down a record of nearly all moderately important events occurring daily is not clear. Whatever the mechanism, if it is composed of rest principle components, it almost certainly uses the self-reinforcing properties of local inhibitory circuits. As discussed in Chapter 10, it also may employ modulating norepinephrine synapses that suppress spontaneous firing but not responses to input.

All our discussion about the cortex has involved inhibitory circuits similar to those provided by basket cells in the hippocampus (i.e., excited by an axon collateral from a large neuron and feeding back on that neuron and its neighbors). There is anatomical evidence that the cortex also contains inhibitory interneurons of the type seen in the olfactory bulb, with dendrodendritic synapses (Schmitt et al., 1976; Shepherd, 1978). Their precise function is unknown, but they should further help to prevent overuse and weakening of connections in the cortex.

The general importance of interneurons in the development of the neocortex is suggested by both phylogeny and ontogeny. The number and proportion of neurons having only local synaptic connections (i.e., interneurons) is highest in the cortex and increases systematically with phylogeny, reaching a peak in humans (see Schmitt et al., 1976). In ontogeny, the interneurons are the last to differentiate in the cortex, and their growth, along with that of the dendritic trees with which they interact, accounts for most of the later enlargement of the cortex.

Not all the cortical interneurons are inhibitory: As in the hippocampus there are excitatory granule cells. It has been hypothesized, because of the large number of them in the neocortex, that they may play an important role in higher cognitive functions. There is little basis for speculating what this role might be, but because of their excitatory action it is possible that they may behave somewhat like the decision module (i.e., maintaining a high degree of plasticity, with the capacity for having their connections both strengthened and weakened). The major factor controlling how their connections are changed, however, might be their success at activating the pyramidal cells rather than external contingencies. For instance, one can imagine their playing a role in solving mental puzzles. The parameters of the puzzle form one set of inputs to the pyramidal cells, priming them for firing. The granule cells then present various patterns of output to the pyramidal cells until one is found that matches the parameters, at which time the pyramidal cells fire and through their inhibitory interneurons reinforce the connections that were involved in producing the solution. Incorrect solutions would be weakened and not remembered, but correct solutions would be protected from weakening by the inhibition.

I find this hypothetical organization very appealing. In effect, the cortex would have tiny rest principle organisms working for it. Instead of trying to solve directly the problems of how to cope with the external world, they would be harnessed for solving the problems set up for them by the cortex. Their reward (rest) would come not from finding food, water, and so on but from finding solutions to the problems.

This proposition breaks down the distinction based on neuronal organization between the basic decision module and the other brain areas. The distinction is further obscured by the use of inhibitory interneurons in the lower brain regions, so that strictly speaking there is no anatomical decision module. The lower brain regions are quite heterogeneous, serving a multitude of functions. Many of these functions are also best served by suppressing plasticity, so it would be advantageous for the organism to supply them with inhibitory interneurons. In many cases this may be genetically determined. In others, it could be at least partially the result of experience. As discussed in earlier chapters, pathways that are frequently used develop inhibitory circuits of various kinds if there are any inhibitory neurons available. This is particularly pronounced if the pathways are able to receive enough rest as the result of external contingencies to become very strong and allow their repeated use, as was the case with the $S_{h+\text{food}} - R_{\text{in}}$ pathway. Such pathways are in effect no longer part of the decision module and bear more resemblance to the higher brain areas with their profuse inhibitory connections. The decision module, therefore, consists of those areas that do not yet have strong self-inhibition, either because anatomically there are not sufficient inhibitory neurons available in the region or because they have not been subjected to the type of experience required for strengthening of inhibitory connections.

I do not mean to imply that most of the brain has become divorced from the rest principle with its inherent "down-plasticity" but only that this property is tempered to varying degrees in many parts. In order to remove this impression further, I would like to correct a misrepresentation I have perpetrated for the sake of simplicity in the preceding discussion. The rest provided by recurrent inhibition and the other inhibitory circuits presented here is almost certainly insufficient to strengthen connections by itself. It merely lessens the amount of weakening enough so that the rest occurring after the stimulus disappears is able to produce a net increase in strength. Under most conditions there is sufficient variability in stimuli for strengthening to occur. Therefore, the general effect of supplying inhibitory interneurons, for instance, in the hippocampal type of neuronal organization, is as I have described: The connections that manage to fire the pyramidal cells become stronger. If the inhibitory circuits were not present, the same input probably would have resulted in a net weakening, but with the inhibition there is, in the long run, a net strengthening.

Evidence that the inhibitory circuits alone are not sufficient for strengthening connections can be seen in both physiological and behavioral results. For instance, in Hubel and Wiesel's studies (1965) a "progressive attenuation of responses" was found in all three areas of the visual cortex with continued presence of the stimulus. Despite various forms of self-inhibition throughout the visual pathways, the cortical cells did not stop firing after the first action potential (i.e., the inhibition merely slowed the rate of responding somewhat, as is also found with Renshaw cell inhibition of motoneurons). During the course of continued stimulation, however, the responding gradually weakened, thus suggesting that the short intervals of rest provided by the inhibitory circuits were insufficient for preventing some weakening of the connections. In agreement with the speculation in Chapter 8 concerning the overuse of sensory pyramids, there was evidence that the weakening occurred at lower levels in the system, because the response of the cortical cell would come back as soon as the stimulus was moved to a new part of the receptive field. On the behavioral side there is the disappearance of the perception of stabilized retinal images and also the various negative afterimages to suggest that weakening occurs with continued use in the visual system.

Therefore, the presence of inhibitory interneurons does not make the pathways follow the *use principle*. There is some evidence, as discussed in Chapter 10, that there is a type of neuronal junction that does create use principle circuits. The inhibitory interneurons we have been discussing here merely shift the emphasis in the rest principle from the requirement for rest to the requirement for use, and they limit the maximal amount of weakening that is likely to occur, so that pathways can continue functioning for longer periods of time and are able to regain whatever strength was lost when a long period of rest finally occurs.

Several brain areas have not been covered in this discussion. In some cases there is good evidence as to the organization, but I have not yet tried to model precisely how these regions would function in a rest principle brain. This is the case with the cerebellum. It is almost entirely inhibitory, with four of the five cell types producing feed-forward inhibition, recurrent lateral inhibition, and recurrent self-inhibition (Eccles, 1967), and with a sixth fiber system involving norepinephrine providing a special type of inhibition. It seems likely that these inhibitory circuits would provide benefits in the cerebellum similar to those seen elsewhere: protecting and reinforcing pathways. Many other brain areas have not been mentioned here because there currently is not enough information for modeling their behavior.

In this chapter we have considered the regional differences in the brain. Chapter 10 covers primarily the temporal differences: arousal states and attention. Inhibitory interneurons are again a central feature of the discussion, partly because of their contribution to these phenomena but also because the requirements of these neurons necessitate sleeping.

10 Sleep, Arousal, and Attention

Inhibitory interneurons provide several very important functions: (1) reducing the signal-to-noise ratio; (2) producing phasic responding and helping to delineate the onset of events; (3) protecting existing connections from weakening with overuse; and (4) contributing to the strengthening of connections that manage to activate them. In this chapter we see also how they can produce a general suppression of firing along all pathways in a given system and how this and the other functions allow them to play a major role in selective attention and memory storage.

These beneficial functions are not obtained without a cost. The inhibitory interneurons also have a requirement: Like all other neurons they need rest. Many of the excitatory neurons get much of their rest as a result of the activity of the inhibitory interneurons, but how can the inhibitory interneurons themselves get enough rest? If each of them received input from only one excitatory neuron, there might be sufficient rest when the excitatory neuron was silent, but often the inhibitory neurons are activated by large numbers of excitatory ones. In addition, as discussed later, there is evidence for either high spontaneous activity or tonic excitatory input to the inhibitory interneurons from sources other than the neurons they inhibit.

Because the functions of the inhibitory interneurons are critical for the normal behaviors of a higher organism, this rest cannot be provided during the animal's daily active period, when it is out in the world searching for food, avoiding predators, and so on and needs to be able to use its full mental capabilities much of the time. Consequently, the animal must find some period each day when it can afford to forego the benefits from its inhibitory interneurons and allow or force them to rest.

Several years ago Evarts (1967) commented on the difficulty in explaining the long time required for sleep in conventional metabolic ways. If neurons are driven to exhaustion by electrical stimulation but given adequate metabolic substrates, they can recover in a matter of minutes. If sleep is needed for replenishing some substrate necessary for the occurrence of the action potential, why, he questioned, do animals need several hours of sleep instead of only a few minutes? A similar argument could be made for the removal of extracellular "waste" products produced during neural activity.

The answer appears to be that the rest is not needed for metabolic reasons but rather for the restoration of synapses. The number of receptors for neural transmitters increases only slowly during rest. In denervation and neural blocking studies, the increase required several days of inactivity. These procedures introduce confounding factors that delay the development or measurement of the increases. The results from metabolic blocking studies bring the time course for increasing the number of receptors down into the same range as the normal duration of sleep. Such a time course was found also for the number of receptors in the pineal gland, which followed the circadian rhythm. It is therefore reasonable that the restoration of receptors in the synapses of the inhibitory interneurons might require several hours of rest every day.

Providing rest for all the inhibitory interneurons is not as simple as it might seem. Consider the visual system in which there are inhibitory interneurons in the retina, in the lateral geniculate nucleus (LGN) relay in the thalamus, and in the cortex (see Singer, 1977). Finding a dark place and closing the eyes may be sufficient for removing most of the excitation to the retinal interneurons and permitting them to rest. The inhibitory neurons in the LGN fire even without excitation from the retina (Singer, 1977), either spontaneously or as the result of tonic facilitory input, and this is likely to be true for the cortical interneurons as well. In order to make them rest, it is therefore necessary to inhibit them directly or to remove the tonic input. Even active inhibition, however, would not be sufficient. There is spontaneous activity in the output neurons of the retina. If the inhibitory interneurons in the LGN are silenced, the relay neurons there transmit the retinal output and add their own spontaneous activity. Consequently, there would be a large excitatory input to the cortical inhibitory interneurons, which certainly would prevent rest to the synapses onto these interneurons and probably also activate the interneurons, despite any general inhibition or absence of tonic excitation, and thus prevent rest for the synapses from the interneurons. In simple terms, the inhibitory interneurons in the LGN and cortex cannot rest at the same time, because making those in the LGN rest increases the excitation to those in the cortex.

The solution to this problem appears to be to let the cortical and LGN interneurons take turns resting. The cortical ones rest first, during slow-wave sleep (or SWS 2, Lidbrink, 1974); then the LGN interneurons rest during paradoxical sleep. The LGN interneurons not only do not rest during slow-wave sleep but instead are overly active. This occurs because the mesencephalic reticular formation (MRF) inhibitory input to the LGN interneurons is removed, thus disinhibiting them (Singer, 1973). As a result, a large inhibitory gradient builds up on the LGN relay neurons that suppresses their spontaneous activity and makes it very difficult for any signal from the retina to get through to the cortex. Consequently, the cortical inhibitory interneurons are allowed to rest with relatively little interference from firing in the optic nerve.

It might be mentioned that although spontaneous activity in the LGN relay neurons is suppressed during slow-wave sleep, it is not abolished. The inhibitory gradient on them periodically decreases, often in phase with the EEG; they then produce synchronous firing as a cluster of action potentials (Singer, 1977). The cause for this spontaneous activity is unclear, but the result would be beneficial for the connections of the cortical interneurons, because it produces infrequent assured use followed by long periods of assured rest, which (as noted in Chapter 9) should produce more strengthening of connections than rest alone.

Eventually the LGN interneurons, which have been overactive in order to let the cortical interneurons rest, have their own turn to rest. With the onset of paradoxical sleep, the MRF inhibitory input that had been silent is now activated, producing a nearly complete suppression of activity in the LGN interneurons (Singer, 1977). The LGN relay neurons, now freed from inhibition, begin spontaneous firing and transmitting of any retinal output. As a result, the cortical cells, other than the inhibitory interneurons, all show an increase in activity (Evarts, 1967), reaching an average level equal to that during wakefulness.

The distribution of interspike intervals from the large cortical neurons can be used as an index of the activity in the cortical inhibitory interneurons. During wakefulness, there is a marked absence of short intervals (Evart, 1967; Steriade, 1978), which would be expected if strong recurrent inhibition prevented the large cells from firing rapidly; the recurrent inhibition stops them from firing immediately after they have just fired. Short intervals appear during slow-wave sleep, suggesting that the functioning of the inhibitory interneurons is suppressed, but because the inputs to the cortex (such as the optic nerve) are generally blocked, the overall level of activity in the large cortical neurons is low. During paradoxical sleep, the short intervals are much more common, apparently as the combined result of the suppressed recurrent inhibition and the unblocked inputs.

Paradoxical sleep in humans is accompanied by dreaming. It seems very likely that the physiological basis for dreams is the cortical activity produced by input from the uninhibited LGN and probably from other sensory relays. The lack of inhibitory control within the cortex may be responsible for the production of taboo themes in dreams, which are suppressed in waking thoughts, but this conclusion probably places too much relevance on the semantic coincidence between neuronal inhibition and behavioral inhibition.

The suggestions regarding the changes in the cortex with sleep can be extended with the model for cortical organization presented in Figure 10.1. This is

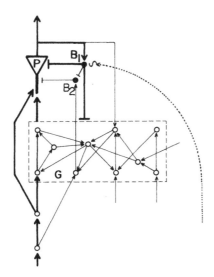

FIG. 10.1.   Proposed model for the local organization within the cerebral cortex.

essentially the same as that for the hippocampus in Chapter 9 (Fig. 9.6), with the following alterations:

1. In that chapter it is shown how the development of expectations would be improved if there were two types of inhibitory neurons, those producing immediate recurrent inhibition (B_1 in Fig. 10.1) and those excited by afferents via granule cells (B_2), and that the former inhibited the latter. This is now incorporated in the model.

2. The network of excitatory granule cells that receive the initial input from the thalamus and then excite the pyramidal cells is now shown in detail within the dashed square in Fig. 10.1. The connections shown are intended only to represent the general complexity and high potential for reverberatory circuits within the granular network. The inhibition from B_1 is seen as acting generally on all the granule cells. (I use the term *granule cell* in order to sustain the analogy with the hippocampal organization, even though it might be more appropriate to call them *stellate cells*.)

3. In line with the finding by Steriade, Deschenes, and Oakson (1974) that the same interneuron may be excited by afferent input and by the firing of pyramidal cells in the cortex, an output from the pyramidal neuron to the granule network is included in the model.

4. The dotted input to B_1 from the midbrain represents the means by which B_1 is made to rest during sleep. It remains to be determined whether this is inhibitory, excitatory, or perhaps due to some neurohumoral substance.

If, as proposed, the activity of B_1 is suppressed during both normal and paradoxical sleep, whereas the input from the thalamus is suppressed only in normal sleep, the changes predicted by the model agree well with recent findings by Steriade (1978) regarding the activity of output neurons and that of interneurons that fired in bursts. Output neurons did not fire in bursts, perhaps because of the immediate recurrent inhibition. B_1, which is fired by P, would, therefore, also be expected not to fire in bursts. In contrast, the granule cells and B_2 in the model would be quite likely to show bursts, first, because they are not subjected to immediate recurrent inhibition and, second, because reverberatory circuits help to fire them.

During sleep, bursting interneurons are freed of the general inhibition from B_1. The effect would be similar to removing the carbon rods from a nuclear reactor: The chain reaction—in this case, reverberation—could proceed unimpeded. During normal sleep, because the input is also removed, the firing rate only doubles; but during dreaming (when rapid eye movements are noted) when input is again present, the firing rate is increased fivefold.

The output neurons show more short intervals between firing in both types of sleep (as discussed earlier), due to the removal of immediate recurrent inhibition from B_1. Delayed recurrent inhibition from B_2 via the granule cells, however, is stronger and lasts longer (from reverberation) during sleep than it does during wakefulness, because both B_2 and the granule cells are free of inhibition from B_1. During normal sleep, the output neurons receive more excitation from the granule cells but less direct input and more inhibition from B_2; consequently, with two out of three factors reducing firing, the output neurons show a slight decrease in activity. However, during dreaming sleep, when there is a large increase in excitation from the granule network plus the presence of direct input from the thalamus, the firing rate of the output neurons is greatly increased to very high levels.

Because of the high rate of firing in both the granule network and the output neurons during dreaming sleep, the connections used will have almost no chance to rest and will not be strengthened. Consequently, there is little or no memory of most dreams. Steriade found, however, that during the first few minutes after awakening there was a nearly complete cessation of firing by large output neurons as well as a sharp reduction in activity by bursting interneurons. Consequently, if one is awakened during a dream, the ensuing rest will allow connections that had just been used, but not yet overused, to become stronger, and portions of the dream may be remembered.

Steriade also found that during arousal, as opposed to quiet wakefulness, there was a nearly complete suppression of spontaneous activity in bursting interneurons and in large (but not small) output neurons. It seems likely that this is at least partially caused by the release of norepinephrine in the cortex during arousal, as discussed later. External signals still get through but evoke less bursting. The result would be that events occurring during arousal would be well remembered, inasmuch as any connection used would be allowed to rest afterward and become stronger.

It is tempting to equate the activity, particularly in the granule network, during quiet wakefulness with thinking, pondering, and daydreaming. The suppression of these mental activities during arousal and orienting would be consistent with the suppression of firing at this time. The relatively high rate of activity in output cells during quiet wakefulness would preclude strengthening of connections onto them. Some strengthening of connections used within the granule network would be possible, but because of the lack of immediate recurrent inhibition within the network the connections could be weakened at a later time. Thus most thoughts or daydreams would leave little memory trace, except in the instances in which they produced arousal. Conceivably, this could be altered, however, by using the B_2 units to provide phasic inhibition to the output cells in certain circumstances to strengthen connections onto them. For instance, finding the solution to a mental puzzle—the "aha!" experience of understanding—might be associated with convergence involving the granule and/or pyramidal cells that would be particularly suited for firing the B_2 units. I must admit that I have no idea how this convergence would be produced, except that it would probably require a more complicated model than that presented here. Nevertheless, in the present model, convergence on B_2 between the afferent input and the axon collateral output could help to distinguish between real signals and spontaneous activity of the pyramidal cells.

One variation on the present model that I find attractive is that instead of having two types of basket cells the functions prescribed to B_1 actually are performed by the small Golgi type II neurons. Because these small neurons operate with only graded potentials, they would not have been observed in studies of action potentials, such as Steriade's. This variation would ascribe four different functions to the four major classes of cells in the cortex. The pyramidal and granule (i.e., stellate) cells would still have the functions described before, but the small Golgi type II neurons would provide tonic inhibition (including immediate recurrent inhibition) of varying degrees depending on the sleep-waking–arousal state, whereas the basket cells would provide phasic inhibition.

Although these suggestions give some idea as to how the cortex, employing the rest principle, could perform the tasks ascribed to it, they are only a beginning. Some features that might be included in more advanced models are: (1) differentiation between types of input (thalamic, intracortical, from other parts of the granule network, and so on); (2) differentiation between types of output (pyramidal, nonpyramidal, subcortical, intracortical, and so on); (3) local control of reverberation within the granule network independent of pyramidal output; (4) local inhibition of portions of the dendritic tree of each pyramidal cell; and (5) the role of possible dendrodendritic or periglomerular-type synapses (Fig. 9.3c, d).

A large amount of research has been devoted to finding the pathways and neural transmitters responsible for controlling the states of arousal. Unfortunately, very little of the evidence at present is conclusive (see Gillin, Mendelson, Sitaram, & Wyatt, 1978). Serotonin, norepinephrine, dopamine, acetylcholine, and specific sleep-factor peptides all have been implicated, but in general it is difficult to determine their precise roles. The least controversial findings are some concerning serotonin. As mentioned earlier, the removal of inhibitory gradients on the LGN relay neurons when desynchronized EEG patterns develop is probably caused by the firing of MRF inputs that inhibit the LGN interneurons. The MRF inputs themselves appear to be cholinergic (see Singer, 1977) and fire during what are called PGO waves or spikes (ponto–geniculo– occipital monophasic negative field potentials). Single-cell recordings in the dorsal raphe nucleus, which is the origin for most of the serotonergic neurons, showed that many units cease firing just before and in temporal association with PGO spikes (McGinty & Harper, 1976). Similarly, electrical stimulation of the raphe nucleus suppresses PGO spikes (Jacobs, Asher, & Dement, 1973). This and other evidence (e.g., Kiianmaa & Fuxe, 1977) tends to confirm the original hypothesis by Jouvet (1972) that serotonergic pathways are important for maintaining slow-wave sleep.

Norepinephrine may be involved in maintaining the EEG desynchronization during wakefulness, but not the behavioral signs of wakefulness, which may be more influenced by dopaminergic neurons (Gillin et al., 1978; Lidbrink, 1974). These results are still inconclusive. Further complicating the question of how sleep and arousal states are produced are the findings of different endogenous compounds that induce sleep (Monnier, Dudler, Gaechter, Maier, Tobler, & Schoewenberger, 1977; Nagasaki, Iriki, & Uchizono, 1976; Pappenheimer, Koski, Fencl, Karnovsky, & Krueger, 1975). Issues concerning the role of circadian pacemakers (Menaker, Takahashi, & Eskin, 1978) and how they interact with the other factors related to sleep still need to be resolved.

I begin the discussion of attention by attacking what for many people may be a "straw man." Several years ago the general view seemed to be that arousal was produced by diffuse excitation supplied by the ascending reticular activating system. There is a classic illustration appearing in many texts showing this system arising from the brainstem and projecting arrows around the brain. To awaken an animal, you stimulated the reticular activating system, which excited neurons around the brain into arousal. Selective attention was then thought to be caused by providing diffuse excitation to the neurons in only one system: To make an animal pay attention to visual stimuli, you excited its visual system.

From a signal-detection viewpoint, these ideas are unreasonable. Imagine that you have two pathways, A and B, coming into the visual cortex, and A has a signal with an intensity of 10 units, whereas B has noise with an intensity of 5 units. The signal-to-noise ratio is 10/5, or 2. To make the animal pay attention to this input, we supply diffuse excitation of, say, 100 units. Pathway A now has 110, B has 105, and the signal-to-noise ratio is 1.05. The more excitation that is added, the lower the ratio becomes, and the harder it is for the animal to detect the signal. Along similar lines, producing arousal by diffuse excitation would be detrimental. The aroused animal would be "senseless."

The diffuse excitation hypothesis also is not supported by the physiological evidence. Ascending pathways providing diffuse excitation have not been found. The ascending norepinephrine pathways would have been the most likely candidates. There is evidence that they are activated during arousal, particularly during important events that require attention (see Cooper, Bloom, & Roth, 1978). They project around the cerebral cortex, the hippocampus, and the cerebellum and influence the large cells in these regions. The norepinephrine in these areas (and in practically all other locations) is not, however, excitatory. Instead, it provides a special kind of inhibition (p. 187).

In place of the diffuse excitation hypothesis, two general hypotheses have developed. Both suggest that attention is controlled by changing the activity of the inhibitory interneurons (Walley & Weiden, 1973; Feeney et al., 1974; Singer, 1977). There is now evidence for the existence of pathways for producing the required diffuse control of the interneurons. As mentioned earlier, the lateral geniculate nucleus has two classes of inhibitory interneurons. Within the LGN are "intrinsic" inhibitory interneurons, providing primarily feed-forward lateral inhibition between the optic nerve pathways. Outside the LGN, in the nucleus reticularis thalami, are inhibitory neurons that apparently receive excitation from axon collaterals of the LGN relay (pathway) neurons and then project back into the LGN, providing relatively diffuse recurrent inhibition on the relay neurons (see Singer, 1977). The latter inhibitory neurons are externally controlled by inputs from the MRF, as mentioned previously, and probably from the frontal eye fields. The intrinsic inhibitory interneurons are externally modulated by output from the visual cortex via corticogeniculate fibers. There are, in fact, as many of these fibers as there are ones going from the LGN to the cortex.

Although both hypotheses postulate controlling attention through the inhibitory interneurons, superficially they appear to be opposites. One states that attention is produced by activating the inhibitory interneurons in the channel from which a signal is expected; the other says that attention is produced by suppressing the inhibitory interneurons in the channel in which there is a signal and activating them in other channels. Despite the apparent contradiction, I think that both hypotheses are likely to be correct; the two methods for controlling attention are merely applied in different situations. I first discuss the methods separately and then present a tentative synthesis.

The hypothesis that lateral inhibition is increased to improve attention is attractive from the signal-detection viewpoint. In the example presented previously, suppose that diffuse excitation were supplied not to the pathways, A and B, but to feed-forward lateral inhibitory neurons between them. Let the strength of the lateral inhibition be L, which is multiplied by the intensity of the input of each pathway and then subtracted from the other pathway. If $L = .4$, the final output of pathway A is $10 - (.4 \times 5) = 8$, and that of B is $5 - (.4 \times 10) = 1$. The signal-to-noise ratio is increased from 2 (when $L = 0$) to 8. Thus increasing the activity of the inhibitory interneurons improves the ability to detect signals. (Notice, however, that this works only for values of L up to .5; if L is increased further, it decreases the signal. If $L = 2$, no signal is received.)

There are various advantages to this method for controlling attention. First, there is no possibility that the diffuse excitation to the lateral inhibitory neurons could be mistaken for a signal. If spontaneous firing happened to occur in one of the excitatory neurons controlling the lateral inhibition, it would merely turn on one or more of the inhibitory interneurons and would not excite the pathway neurons. Second, the diffuse excitation to lateral inhibitory interneurons could be rather indiscriminate; it does not matter much if it is a bit stronger to one interneuron than to another. For instance, if L was .4 for the neuron inhibiting A and .3 for the one inhibiting B, the final outputs are 8 and 2, the signal-to-noise ratio is changed slightly, but the signal still gets through with little atleration. Third, as long as the strength of L is not changed too dramatically, the intensity of the final signal is not changed very much. Finally, if the neurons employ the rest principle, the efficiency of memory storage increases at the same time and in the same modality as attention. There are various ways in which increasing the activity of inhibitory interneurons increases memory storage, some of which were discussed in the preceding section on sleep. In the example here, with lateral inhibition, a pathway is forced to rest after the signal is removed if inhibition is high, because noise in that pathway is suppressed by lateral inhibition from the pathway that now has the signal. The rest, of course, strengthens the connections previously used and creates a memory of the preceding signal. By linking memory storage to attention, it would be possible to reserve more space in the brain for storing important information (i.e., that occurring jointly with attention) by not wasting space storing all the information impinging on the organism.

There is experimental evidence supporting this hypothesis. Evoked potential recordings showed indications of increased inhibition in the channels through which important information was expected (Young, Ellison, & Feeney, 1971). Arousal also was found to increase the recurrent inhibition in the visual cortex and midsuprasylvian association cortex (Pittman & Feeney, 1974), but to decrease it in the motor cortex (Feeney et al., 1974). A decrease also was found in the LGN, which seems somewhat in conflict with the hypothesis.

The other general hypothesis emphasizes the ability of inhibitory interneurons to block activity in pathways or in whole modalities. As seen in the earlier example, if the lateral inhibition is made strong enough, output from all pathways in the system can be prevented. We also saw how this was accomplished in the LGN during slow-wave sleep and drowsy wakefulness to block input to the cortex along the optic nerve.

There is good behavioral evidence that selective blocking of separate modalities can occur with attention. For instance, paying attention to one modality increases the threshold for perceiving stimuli in other modalities (see Treisman, 1969). On the physiological level, during intense attention to auditory stimuli, the excitability of the LGN is reduced (Horn & Wiesenfeld, 1974). One route that has been suggested as a means for modulating LGN excitability with selective attention is a functional pathway from the frontal eye fields to the perigeniculate nucleus of the nucleus reticularis thalami (Tsumoto & Suzuki, 1976). Stimulation of the frontal eye fields causes inhibition of the cells in this nucleus that otherwise produce recurrent inhibition onto the LGN relay neurons; the stimulation, therefore, results in the removal of inhibition from the LGN relay cells and allows signals to pass more easily. It will be remembered that this is the same way that the MRF regulated excitability of the LGN, through the rather diffuse recurrent inhibition neurons (as distinct from the intrinsic inhibitory circuits within the LGN). The influence of the frontal eye fields does not go through the MRF but merely terminates on the same thalamic nucleus.

Singer (1977) has suggested a model for controlling binocular inputs, in which the intrinsic inhibitory circuits in the LGN also act in accordance with this hypothesis. The net effect of the model is to increase the ability to see objects on the horopter (i.e., the loca. h in space from which visual signals strike corresponding retinal areas and thus are seen as one stimulus, whereas points off the horopter are seen doubly.)

From physiological studies it is known that each corticogeniculate fiber projects to the LGN column that excites it. In the LGN these fibers apparently produce excitatory synapses onto inhibitory interneurons and also onto the relay neurons. Singer hypothesizes that they do not really innervate the intrinsic inhibitory interneurons but rather synapse on special inhibitory neurons that inhibit the intrinsic inhibitory interneurons: Firing of the fibers thus reduces inhibition on the relay cells. In the model, a stimulus on the horopter produces inputs from both eyes onto the same LGN column and then onto the cortex, where it is able to excite the corticogeniculate fiber and thereby remove inhibition in that column. Consequently, the horopter stimulus henceforth passes more easily through the LGN, whereas stimuli off the horopter are faced with increased inhibition in their LGN columns. Singer concludes that in addition to binocular vision: "it is tempting to assume that for other aspects of visual information also the LGN is serving as an 'internal retina' from which the cortex chooses through its efferent projections in a highly selective way those items that are relevant in a particular phase of image processing."

Unfortunately, it is not possible to state how the cortex selects the other aspects. There are three other types of intrinsic inhibition in the LGN (in addition to that between the inputs from the two eyes), serving to increase contrasts between adjacent retinal fields, between "on" and "off" responses, and between transient and sustained afferent systems. Unlike the binocular system, these three systems, which all deal with contrasts, have an optimal level of inhibition that produces the most signal and the least noise: Complete removal of inhibition from them would decrease the chances of detecting signals. Consequently, Singer's model would not work for these systems.

There are various ways to avoid this contradiction:

1. Perhaps the purpose of the corticogeniculate fibers is to remove the signals that stimulate them. This would help delineate the onset of stimuli, in a way similar to the intrinsic inhibition between "on" and "off" responses. Redundant

firing is avoided. The binocular system would act similarly if it were really a disparity detector for gauging depth.

2. All four systems would operate like Singer's model if the level of intrinsic inhibition were maintained always above the optimal point.

3. There may be no single mode of action for the corticogeniculate fibers. They are characterized by a high degree of heterogeneity as to what activates them and their transmission rate, so perhaps they also differ as to how they affect the LGN.

4. The other three systems might operate in accordance with Singer's model if each corticogeniculate fiber acted selectively to remove only incoming inhibition onto its relay cell and not outgoing inhibition onto other relay cells.

5. The evidence for concluding that corticogeniculate fibers decrease inhibition in the LGN is controversial, and some of it easily could be interpreted as showing that the fibers increase the intrinsic inhibition. For instance, the finding that stimulation of a particular cortical cell causes excitation in the LGN relay neurons projecting to it but inhibition to relay neurons projecting to adjacent cortical cells might be explained in this way. The cortical cell excites the lateral inhibitory neurons originating in its LGN column, thus increasing inhibition to all adjacent columns. Suppressing firing in the adjacent columns then reduces the inhibition coming back onto the first column, which in conjunction with the direct synapses of the fibers onto the LGN relay cells causes an excitation in the LGN column projecting to the stimulated cortical cell. If the corticogeniculate fibers increase LGN intrinsic inhibition, they would increase the signals to themselves, so long as the inhibition did not get too high, from the three contrast systems and from the binocular system if it acts as a disparity detector.

This interpretation avoids having to postulate special inhibitory neurons juxtaposed between the corticogeniculate fibers and the LGN intrinsic inhibitory interneurons, which Singer needed to change the excitatory output of the fibers into inhibition. This interpretation is no longer in accordance with the second hypothesis for attention but rather with the first.

There currently is not enough evidence for deciding which, if any, of the foregoing suggestions is correct. Nevertheless, it seems safe to conclude that the corticogeniculate fibers play a role in selective attention within the visual system by interacting with the intrinsic inhibitory interneurons in the LGN to affect the signals reaching the cortex.

In summary, there is evidence that attention involves small increases in inhibition sufficient to raise the signal-to-noise ratio (Method 1), and there is also evidence that attention involves large increases in inhibition sufficient to suppress all output from some systems, while perhaps concomitantly decreasing inhibition in another system (Method 2). How can both be true?

Part of the discrepancy between the two methods arises merely from different vantage points. The example given for Method 1 involved two pathways, *A* and

B, and for attention the lateral inhibition was optimally increased to the point where the noise from *B* was eliminated. Now suppose that *A* and *B* are two modalities, and we again apply Method 1, increasing the lateral inhibition between the modalities sufficiently to produce the maximum signal-to-noise ratio. Hypothetically this requires that all output from *B* is suppressed. The easiest way to do this would be through the inhibitory interneurons between the pathways in modality *B*, increasing their activity enough so that there is no output from *B*. This is, of course, Method 2. Applying Method 1 between systems is best effected by applying Method 2 within the systems. The removal of some inhibition from *A* could occur automatically if any recurrent inhibition is present, inasmuch as suppressing *B* removes its recurrent inhibiton on *A* or, more precisely, removes its excitation of the inhibitory interneurons within *A*.

Although this solution may explain the discrepancy in some situations, it is too simple, and there are real differences between the two methods. For instance, in the foregoing example, Method 2 would suggest that modality *A* should optimally be freed of all inhibition, whereas Method 1 suggests that the inhibition in *A* should be maintained at a moderate level.

A more complete solution visualizes both methods as being employed in different situations. For instance, the poor attention found during a quiet relaxed period may be the result of low levels of inhibition in all systems (Method 1). Anticipation of a signal increases the inhibition toward the optimal level in the system in which the signal is expected. If a signal of some kind is expected, but the channel is unknown, the inhibition could be increased toward optimal in all systems likely to receive the signal (Method 1). Once the organism begins receiving the signal, the inhibition in the other systems is increased to very high levels, thus suppressing their outputs (Method 2).

The initial reception of the signal might play an important role in producing the high inhibition in the other systems. This would be analogous to the situation at the level of individual neurons. External inputs related to attention increase the activity in the inhibitory interneurons between *A* and *B* only slightly. Strong inhibition of *B* occurs only when the signal to *A* arrives and combines with the external input to excite the inhibitory interneurons.

It is also possible that different inhibitory systems may be used preferentially for the two methods. For example, the diffuse recurrent inhibition from the nucleus reticularis thalami to the LGN would be ill-suited for modulating inhibition between low and moderate levels with Method 1, because the increases in inhibition it provides do little to increase the signal-to-noise ratio from the LGN; its diffuse inhibition, however, is very well suited for the general suppression of LGN output needed by Method 2.

It has been mentioned already how Method 1 would correlate memory storage with attention. Method 2 also could have a role in memory, which has been alluded to in earlier chapters. When an organism is involved in an activity that provides a signal X to one system and then a signal Y to a second system, the inhibition of the first system when Y is present would help to strengthen the connections that had been fired by X. In Chapter 8 this was suggested as occurring with the verbal and imagery systems: A word that stimulated the verbal system and then evoked activity in the visual imagery system, thus causing high inhibition of the verbal system, would be better remembered than one that did not evoke an image. Such interactions might also involve motor systems as well as the sensory systems.

The catecholamines, norephinephrine (NE) and dopamine (DA), have been implicated in attention (Mantovani, Bartolini, & Pepeu, 1977; Matthysse, 1977; Rolls, 1975) and in memory (Grossman, 1977; Mason & Fibiger, 1978; Mora, 1977). This is, of course, not surprising, because the catecholamines have also been implicated in practically all other activities. As stated earlier, this is partly because of the improved tools for studying these substances and may attest only to the degree of interdependence found in the brain, such that any change in one system is likely to be reflected in all other systems. Nevertheless, the evidence relating the catecholamines to attention and memory appears to be particularly strong.

There has been an unfortunate tendency in the past to categorize all transmitters as either excitatory or inhibitory and then to treat all the excitatory ones as being equivalent to one another and all the inhibitory ones as being equivalent. The current physiological evidence suggests that this is a gross oversimplification: NE, for instance, does not produce the same postsynaptic effects as GABA. This bimodal categorizing has probably been quite detrimental to the development of an understanding of how the nervous system actually functions. I would like to try a different approach, starting with the little clear evidence we do have as to the effects of NE and DA and suggesting how these modulators (not transmitters) might be specifically employed for the benefit of a rest principle brain.

From the physiological evidence, a very interesting role for NE in memory storage would be predicted in a brain employing the rest principle. NE-releasing neurons project throughout the cerebral cortex, the hippocampus, and the cerebellar cortex (see Bloom, 1975), producing effects on the large pyramidal and Purkinje cells. The actions on the Purkinje cells in the cerebellum have been studied most thoroughly. There appear to be enough NE fibers so that every Purkinje cell is innervated.

Application of NE or stimulation of NE fibers causes an unusual postsynaptic reaction in the Purkinje cells. It selectively suppresses their spontaneous firing but has no effect on their firing in response to afferent input, and according to Bloom (1975) it "specifically augments the population of long pauses." Similar effects are found in the hippocampus. That NE acts as a modulator rather than as a transmitter is supported by the finding that NE fibers in the cortex seldom form real synapses; the NE released may diffuse instead around the large cells, somewhat like a local hormone, thus causing a widespread general effect (Descarries, Watkins, & Lapierre, 1977).

The rest principle would predict that NE would greatly enhance the strengthening of connections in these structures and thus the storage of memory. Normally these large cells show a fair amount of spontaneous activity. Consequently, firing produced by a true signal is liable to be followed by spontaneous activity that would prevent the connections from resting and being strengthened. By selectively removing spontaneous activity and increasing the long pauses, NE would not interfere with the responding to signals but would help to assure that rest would follow use and that the connections used therefore would grow stronger.

The acquisition of NE inputs to these structures is similar to the acquisition of the inhibitory interneurons in that it helps prevent the weakening of connections and thus increases the chances of their being strengthened. The effect of NE differs from that of the inhibitory interneurons, most of which probably release GABA, and helps to solve a problem. With the usual inhibition, after a moderate level has been reached, there is a trade-off between the ability to store memories and the ability to maintain signal intensity and detect weaker signals; if the inhibition is increased further to allow more rest and better memory storage, the output-signal intensity is likely to be reduced and only strong stimuli will be perceived. In an emergency situation, for instance, this would be detrimental. The animal should record the events as well as possible, but at the same time it should respond vigorously and not have its stimulus input suppressed. It might be noted that the problem may not have been solved completely and may cause a narrowing of the range of stimuli perceived and perhaps incapacitation in an emergency. Nevertheless, NE input helps to prevent this problem because the inhibition is selective: Signals are not impaired, but only the noise of spontaneous firing.

We might ask why the large neurons were not designed without spontaneous activity in the first place. There probably are several advantages to be gained from their having spontaneous activity, such as allowing more freedom and variability of behavior when nothing important has to be done. An advantage related to the rest principle is that it is more economical to have spontaneous activity prevent the strengthening of connections much of the time. As mentioned earlier, this could contribute to the failure to store memories during sleep. The existence of spontaneous activity and a specific system, NE inputs, for removing it allows the brain to choose whether or not to record memories. In particular, the NE neurons in the central nervous system are activated by acute stress (see Cooper et al., 1978). This should cause the hippocampus, cerebral cortex, and cerebellum to be in a state for optimal recording of information during such situations. The NE input would amount to the "now print" mechanism that Livingston (1967) speculated the brain should contain. It would be advantageous if the NE "now print" system could be activated at times when stimuli related to the removal of physiological needs were received (as seems to be the case, see Rolls, 1975) and when novel stimuli were presented (as Livingston had suggested), and if the NE output to the various higher brain areas could be selectively activated to help print memories in specific modalities alone.

By an odd coincidence, while I was writing the preceding paragraphs, a report came to my desk showing that Korsakoff's syndrome is associated with low levels of brain NE activity (McEntee & Mair, 1979). Korsakoff's syndrome is specifically characterized by an inability to remember recent events. The degree of memory impairment shows a strong negative correlation ($r = -.83$) with the amount of the principal NE metabolite, used as an indicatory for NE activity.

This view of NE as increasing the chances that connections will be strengthened, together with the discussion about happiness at the end of Chapter 8, produces predictions in agreement with the "catecholamine theory for affective disorders" (Cooper et al., 1978; Sandler, Ruthven, Goodwin, Reynolds, Rao, & Coppen, 1979). If for some reason NE synapses were less active, there would be fewer connections being strengthened. Because there seems to be a perfect correlation between the net amount of strengthening occurring and the feeling of happiness, a reduction in NE activity would reduce the general level of happiness. The catecholamine theory (Cooper et al., 1978) states that: "In general, behavioral depression may be related to a deficiency of catecholamine (usually norepinephrine) at functionally important central adrenergic synapses." The theory is based upon findings that drugs that increase the supply of NE available at receptors are effective in treating depression, whereas reserpine, which depletes NE can cause depression.

Although NE may have a more general affect on the number of connections being strengthened, it certainly is not the only transmitter/modulator that has an effect. Consequently, NE deficiency would not be the only possible cause of depression. This is in agreement with recent findings suggesting that DA, histamine, octopamine, tyramine, and other substances may play a role in maintaining affect (Sandler et al., 1979).

Dopamine is closely related to NE; it is a precursor from which NE is made, and as with NE there are ascending DA bundles starting in the brainstem but, with the exception of the frontal cortex, having projections terminating in subcortical regions. The only place where the actions of DA synapses have been studied in detail lies outside the brain, in the sympathetic ganglia. At least here, DA does not act as a simple transmitter but has unusual effects.

In the sympathetic ganglia, excitatory input neurons, releasing acetylcholine, make two types of synapses onto each of their target cells: nicotinic synapses that produce fast excitatory postsynaptic potentials and are responsible for firing the postsynaptic cell, and muscarinic synapses producing a slow excitatory postsynaptic potential, which makes it easier for the nicotinic synapses to activate the target. The input neurons also excite small "SIF" interneurons, which then release DA onto the target cells. DA produces a slow inhibitory postsynaptic potential that apparently suppresses activity for a short time in the target cell. The cAMP produced within the target cell as a result of DA then causes an enhancement of the muscarinic slow excitatory postsynaptic potential that lasts for very long periods of time, in extreme cases up to 3 hours, and makes the target easier to fire during this time.

Like GABA and NE, DA in this arrangement would circumvent the weakening of connections with overuse from the rest principle, but DA goes even further. It makes the junction act for a while according to the use principle. Use of the junction makes it easier for the junction to be used again, for as long as the cAMP is still having an influence. Because the synapse exciting the DA neuron and the synapse at which DA is released are still probably controlled by the rest principle, there still would be the potential for weakening the junction, but it would require extremely long overuse, weakening first the synapses of the DA neuron and then the acetylcholine synapses (Kobayashi et al., 1978; Libet, 1977; Perkins, 1975).

Such constructed use principle junctions would be beneficial in many circuits. During an emergency situation it would be advantageous to be able to provide continual vigorous activation to various organs. This, however, would require firing rates that would rapidly weaken normal circuits; without DA, high levels of activation could be maintained only for short periods of time before the neural circuits gave out. With the DA junctions, use does not weaken but strengthens pathways, so the vigorous activation could easily be maintained for the duration of the emergency.

Circuits containing DA junctions could be used for short-term storage of information. The pathways used during the input of the information would remain easier to fire while the cAMP was still effective. Consequently, they could readily be traversed again during this period for retrieval of the information.

DA junctions would be very useful in circuits producing slow movements, such as reaching for small objects. Such movements involve two opposing systems (e.g., one activating extensor muscles and the other, flexor muscles) and require that both systems be activated at the same time to different degrees, so that the flexor system provides opposition to the extension, slowing and smoothing the action and providing time for small corrections to be made during the course of the movement. Weakening with use, and particularly the faster weakening of the more active system, would prevent the production of such slow smooth movements with normal circuits. Either uncoordinated sporadic outputs or oscillatory outputs from the two systems would be expected, depending on the amount of inhibition coupling the systems. All the solutions previously mentioned for counteracting this weakening would interfere with the required continual activation or would be effective only for all-or-none movements in which only one of the two systems is active. The DA junctions, however, prevent weakening without producing too much interference with the rate of firing and consequently would allow slow smooth movements. This, however, would require rather fine tuning of the DA activity. In the DA junctions in the ganglia, use causes a strengthening, which also would be detrimental to the movements. Consequently, either the DA output would have to be limited so that it only offset the weakening in the acetylcholine synapses in the junctions or the DA junctions would have to be interspersed with normal excitatory synapses so that the strengthening in the former just offset the weakening in the latter. If for some reason the DA activity were reduced, smooth slow movements would again be prevented. Furthermore, because continued high output would be impossible, muscle strength would be limited, particularly for tasks requiring prolonged exertion. Such symptoms are found in Parkinson's disease, which is caused apparently by some deficiency in the DA neurons; the symptoms can be removed by administration of L-dopa, the precursor of DA.

The inclusion of DA junctions also would improve the ability to concentrate on one stimulus or idea for a long time. With no inhibition, any circuit used will weaken rapidly, and some other pathway with greater strength will then be used. The inclusion of recurrent GABA inhibition will slow the rate of use so a pathway will fire less frequently and therefore weaken more slowly, but it would not prevent the weakening. The lateral components of the inhibition will suppress some competitive pathways, but the point still will be reached when they are stronger than the pathway being used. NE synapses could further delay the switching to other pathways but, again, could not stop it. Only the DA junctions that not only prevent weakening but actually cause strengthening with use would allow long-term repetitive use. It seems likely that this may be related to the difficulty that patients with Parkinson's disease have with concentrating and remaining alert, problems also corrected with L-dopa. Depletion of DA in animals interferes with any complex learned behavior that requires long-term use of some circuits (Grossman, 1977; Mantovani et al., 1977). It also has been found that depletion of DA interferes with internal initiation of behavior but not with reflexive actions, perhaps because only the former requires repetitive firing in an internal "planning circuit."

DA is not entirely beneficial. As we see throughout this book, the use principle generally is detrimental to behavior. Development of use principle DA junctions creates the potential for the same type of problems that have been predicted for use principle organisms. If too much DA activity is present, the person would be expected to behave like the use principle push-me–pull-you modeled in Chapter 1: He would become stuck on one response or one idea. The same response or response cycle might be emitted for hours on end. Ideas not dependent on external stimuli would turn into obsessions. The more often the thought pattern is repeated, the stronger it would become, until the person might find it difficult to think of anything else. Even the DA junctions have limits and probably can be weakened with too rapid input, so very short length reverberating circuits would not be a problem as they would be in a pure use principle organism. The DA junctions instead would tend to "get stuck" on somewhat longer reverberating pathways. Consequently, the high DA organism would tend to show repetitive response cycles ($A, B, C, A, B, C, A, \ldots$) rather than merely continuing the same response ($A, A, A, \ldots$) and would not get stuck pushing against a wall but rather on a cycle such as pacing back and forth. Similarly, the obsessions would tend to involve relatively complex repetitive patterns (e.g., I am afraid because they are out to get me because I am afraid because they . . .) rather than a single thought component (e.g., I, I, I, . . .). As discussed in the next section, there are reasons for speculating that the obsessions produced by use principle circuits will include the component "I."

In less severe cases, when weakening of the DA junctions begins at a lower rate of firing (but still much higher than in normal organisms), the response cycles or obsessive thought patterns would involve even more complex and longer reverberating circuits. The activity in the circuits, however, could be more easily interrupted by external stimuli than in the severe cases. Nevertheless, any neural activity that managed to excite a component of the reverberating circuit would be likely to reinstate the repetitive response cycle or obsessive thought. The individual also would find it difficult, but probably not impossible, to stop the activity in the reverberating circuit by trying, for instance, to concentrate on some other thought.

Also in these less severe cases it often would be possible to destroy the reverberating circuit. To do this it would be necessary to increase the firing rate in the circuit above that chosen by the circuit itself and to maintain this high rate of activity for a prolonged period of time. The person should be presented with as many stimuli as possible having inputs to the reverberating circuit and should be instructed to concentrate on the obsession rather than trying to block it. As suggested earlier, such excessive use first will weaken the synapses of the DA neurons; once this line of defense is removed, the excitatory connections in the junctions can be fired even more rapidly (because the inhibitory effect of DA also is removed) and quickly weakened. From the correlation between the net strengthening (minus weakening) and happiness, it would be expected that this should be an unpleasant experience, particularly once the DA defenses are removed and the rapid weakening of the excitatory connections occurs. Unfortunately, if the development of the first reverberatory circuit was due to a physiological disorder causing a general excess of DA activity, it is quite likely that other reverberatory circuits would develop in the future.

These speculations are based upon how the DA junction seen in ganglia would act in a brain otherwise employing the rest principle. (If all synapses employed the use principle, there would be nothing unique about the DA junctions and no reason to relate them to such bizarre behaviors.) There are grounds for questioning these bases. Such DA junctions have not yet been identified in the brain itself. And there is the central question of the validity of the rest principle and the generality of it for all other connections. Nevertheless, there is rather strong evidence for the conclusions.

Animals given dopaminergic drugs or treated in ways to increase the responsivity to DA do show extreme stereotypic behaviors, involving response cycles that may continue for long periods of time. Drugs that block DA receptors stop the stereotypic behaviors.

In humans, the "dopaminergic hypothesis for schizophrenia" has gained a large amount of support. "Getting stuck" is, of course, a typical characteristic of schizophrenia, and both repetitive response cycles and obsessive thought patterns are observed. Administration of dopaminergic drugs to schizophrenics often intensifies the symptoms. Of more practical importance, drugs that block DA receptors relieve the symptoms. Such drugs, called *neuroleptics,* have created the "modern revolution in psychiatry." Administration of neuroleptics, such as haloperidol, does allow obsessive thoughts to disappear (Matthysse, 1977), as would be expected, inasmuch as this would remove the use principle effect of the DA junctions, and the reverberating circuits could weaken normally with overuse. The conclusions as to how obsessions could be removed experientially without drugs and the problem of how new obsessions would be likely to develop are in accordance with the results obtained by earlier psychiatric treatments such as psychotherapy.

It is, of course, quite possible that disorders with substances other than DA are involved in schizophrenia or some kinds of schizophrenia. DA may not be the only modulator creating use principle junctions; it would not be at all surprising to find, for instance, that NE also had this effect. There also may be specific systems for controlling the DA activity, and disorders in these systems rather than DA per se may be responsible for schizophrenia. I should also caution that even if the speculations here about DA and NE do turn out to be true, they may apply only to certain populations of these neurons. Both the DA and NE neurons constitute heterogeneous groups. New evidence suggests two types of DA receptors (Costall & Naylor, 1976; Katz, 1979) and may argue strongly against the ideas I presented about Parkinson's disease, if the suggestions are confirmed that the DA receptor involved in the disease does not cause the production of cAMP.

I conclude with a brief speculative comment on the most speculative question in the realm of psychology, the origin of consciousness, and suggest how it might benefit from one part of the brain's operating according to the rest principle, a second part according to a limited use principle, and a third part recording in a rather neutral way the inputs from the first two parts. Consciousness often has been thought to be dependent on an awareness of one's self, plus an awareness of everything else that is not one's self, and a clear distinction between the two. The only feature completely differentiating the self from other things is permanence: All other things are gone sometimes, but the self is always present. Consequently, stimuli for other things are not always available and, if available, may disappear; but some stimuli (e.g., somatosensory input and cumulative input from large regions of the brain itself) are always available and can be maintained indefinitely.

Distinct *rest* and *use* principle systems would aid in separating these two classes (transient and permanent) of inputs and therefore in associating members within each class and developing the required *self* and *other things* concepts. This would be so because the rest principle system will relay transients (which have strengthened connections) and not permanent signals (which have weakened connections), whereas the use principle system preferentially will relay permanent signals (which have strengthened connections).

The cortex, therefore, will receive the two types of inputs from anatomically different sources and perhaps projecting to different cortical locations. To the extent that the two systems can be independently activated, there also will be a temporal separation between the two types of inputs. This spatial and perhaps temporal segregation will facilitate greatly the formation of associations, the development of "concept" neurons for each of the two types of inputs, and the distinction between them. Memories are likely to be labeled as being related to the systems if either the systems project to different cortical areas or the storage involves strengthening not only of intracortical connections but also of input and output connections. The output from the concept neurons for self cannot maintain connections on the rest principle system because of their lack of transience but would evoke strong responses in the use principle system. Because this system projects preferentially to the concept neurons for self, this creates a reverberatory circuit and the preoccupation of a large percentage of the use principle connections with the self. Consequently, as discussed earlier, obsessive ideas would be expected to contain components related to self.

A creature with the proposed brain organization, therefore, would be almost certain to develop a concept or awareness of itself, a distinct awareness of things other than itself, a set of memories designated as pertaining to itself, another set of memories designated as pertaining to other things, and a system preoccupied with matters concerning the self and capable of dwelling at length on these matters. The role that these factors play in consciousness depends on how it is defined, and there appears to be no generally accepted definition for consciousness (Natsoulas, 1978). Nevertheless, the importance of self-awareness for consciousness is widely accepted (Jaynes, 1976); the role of self-memories for self-awareness can be ascertained from studies of patients with amnesia; Jaynes and others have stressed the necessity for the ability to think about one's self; and some developmental psychologists have emphasized the importance of the self–other distinction for the emergence of consciousness. The difficulty in defining consciousness and much of the confusion about it probably stems from the fact that it can be viewed only by introspection. Consequently, the only proper conclusion I can make is that these factors appear to form a sufficient basis for what I call, in myself, "consciousness"; only you can specify the role they play for your consciousness.

While writing this book and presenting the ideas to colleagues, I have commonly had to face two philosophical objections. The first comes from a belief that reductionism is impossible in psychology. It has been very disconcerting to have a philosopher tell me, after I had just completed what seemed to me an adequate and satisfying reductionistic explanation for some psychological phenomenon, that what I had done was impossible and that therefore I had not done it. I have thus been led to the conclusion that the tools of philosophy must be inadequate for determining a priori whether reductionism will be impossible for psychological results and that the only way to see whether reductionism works in this field is to try it. Monod (1972) had a stronger reply to this type of objection:

> According to these holist schools which, phoenixlike, spring anew with every generation, only failure awaits attempts to reduce the properties of a very complex organization to the "sum" of the properties of its parts. A most foolish and wrongheaded quarrel it is, merely testifying to the "holists'" profound misappreciation of scientific method and of the crucial role analysis plays in it. If a Martian engineer were trying to understand one of our earthling computers, how far could he conceivably get were he, on principle, to refuse to dissect the basic electronic components which in the machine execute the operations of propositional algebra? [p. 79].

The second objection is to general theories in psychology: No single theory could be expected to explain more than a small set of the diverse phenomena found in the field. This certainly would not be true, however, for a theory based upon a new, correct specification of the rules governing neuronal plasticity (i.e., the changes in the strength of neural connections). In Monod's example, knowledge about the basic components is necessary for an understanding of computers. Similarly, a knowledge of plasticity rules is a necessary prerequisite for an understanding, at least at a physiological level, of nearly all phenomena in psychology.

In both the computer and the nervous system, knowledge about the basic components is necessary, but it is not sufficient. There are also other factors that must be known. I believe, however, that for many cases in psychology these other factors already have been determined. Thus all that has been missing has been the understanding of plasticity. Consequently, if the rest principle is a correct description of the rules for plasticity, it must of necessity explain a wide range of phenomena; if it were unable to do so, this would be prima facie evidence that the rest principle was not correct.

On the other hand, there is a larger set of psychological phenomena in which the remaining factors have not yet been established. For instance, the model given in this volume for the cellular organization in the cortex is certainly incomplete, and because many of the missing details probably are genetically determined, we cannot hope to derive them from the rules for plasticity. Consequently, at present, knowing how plasticity works cannot produce a complete understanding of cortical functions.

The correct rules for plasticity, nevertheless, would be very useful in the search for the missing factors affecting cortical functions and all other unexplained psychological phenomena, helping to guide researchers to look for the right factors and to recognize that they are correct when they are found. In the past, the only simple rule for plasticity has been the use principle, which, as we have seen, is almost certainly wrong. Consequently, it seems likely that there have been instances when scientists have properly uncovered all the correct "nonplasticity" factors for explaining results, but because these factors did not work when combined with the use principle, the scientists did not realize that they had the correct factors. The general failure to produce reasonable models for brain functions can, I believe, be traced primarily to the previous reliance upon the use principle. The rest principle at least offers an alternative set of rules for plasticity and thus provides an additional way of thinking for individuals trying to make such models.

The question remains whether the rest principle represents the correct rules for plasticity. At a detailed level, the answer clearly must be "no." First, the rest principle is inadequate because of the parameters left unspecified: The issue of which of the models presented in Table 3.2 are correct must be resolved; the time courses for strengthening and weakening connections remain to be determined. Second, there are probably many complications, modifications, and variations of the rest principle rules that have evolved in the nervous system. Inhibition of a pathway well may produce more strengthening of the connections than rest alone, perhaps as a result of the cyclic AMP produced by inhibitory transmitters and modulators, as is suggested by the work with the dopamine junctions. The exact rules for plasticity probably also differ somewhat for different types of synapses: One set of physiological mechanisms may be more important for changing the strength of serotonergic synapses, another set for cholinergic synapses, and so on.

As a first approximation, however, the rest principle is, I believe, correct. For most applications, this should be adequate for producing a reasonably good explanation for behavior, once the other, nonplasticity, factors are identified. Hopefully, this therefore could represent the beginning for a new era for psychology, a period when it will become firmly based on neurophysiology and can rightfully take its place among the sciences.

References

Aghajanian, G. K., & Bunney, B. S. Central dopaminergic neurons: Neurophysiological identification and responses to drugs. In E. Usdin & S. M. Snyder (Eds.), *Frontiers in catecholamine research*. Oxford: Pergamon, 1973.

Almon, R. R., Andrew, C. G., & Appel, S. H. Acetylcholine receptors in normal and denervated slow and fast muscle. *Biochemistry*, 1974, *13*, 5522-5528.

Andersen, P. Organization of hippocampal neurons and their interconnections. In R. L. Isaacson & K. H. Pribram (Eds.), *The hippocampus 1*. New York: Plenum, 1975.

Andersen, P., Eccles, J. C., & Loyning, Y. Recurrent inhibition in the hippocampus with identification of the inhibitory cell and its synapses. *Nature*, 1963, *198*, 540-542.

Andersen, P., Gross, G. N., Lømo, T., & Sveen, O. Participation of inhibitory and excitatory interneurones in the control of hippocampal output. In M. A. B. Brazier (Ed.), *The interneuron*. Berkeley: University of California, 1969.

Annunziato, L., & Moore, K. E. Increased ability of apomorphine to reduce serum concentrations of prolactin in rats treated chronically with alpha-methyltyrosine. *Life Sciences*, 1977, *21*, 1845-1850.

Appel, S. H., Roses, A. D., Almon, R. R., Andrew, C. G., Smith, P. B., McNamara, J. O., & Butterfield, D. A. Membrane biochemical approaches to altered muscle structure and function. In R. O. Brady (Ed.), *The nervous system. Vol. 1: The basic neurosciences*. New York: Raven, 1975.

Aurbach, G. O., Fedak, S. A., Woodward, C. J., Palmer, J. S., Hauser, D., & Troxer, F. Beta-adrenergic receptor: Stereospecific interaction of iodinated beta-blocking agent with high affinity site. *Science*, 1974, *186*, 1223-1224.

Axelsson, J., & Thesleff, S. A study of supersensitivity in denervated mammalian skeletal muscle. *Journal of Physiology* (London), 1959, *147*, 178-192.

Azrin, N. H. Punishment of elicited aggression. *Journal of the Experimental Analysis Behaviour* 1970, *14*, 7-10.

Azrin, N. H., & Holz, W. C. Punishment. In W. K. Honig (Ed.), *Operant behavior: Areas of research and application*. New York: Appleton-Century-Crofts, 1966.

Ball, G. G. Electrical self-stimulation of the brain and sensory inhibition. *Psychonomic Science*, 1967, *8*, 489-490.

Bar, R. S., Gorden, P., Roth, J., Kahn, C. R., & DeMeyts, P. Fluctuation in the affinity and concentration of insulin receptors on circulating monocytes of obese patients: Effects of starvation, refeeding and dieting. *Journal of Clinical Investigation*, 1976, *58*, 1123-1135.

Barnes, G. W., & Kish, G. B. On some properties of visual reinforcement. *American Psychologist*, 1958, *13*, 417.

Barondes, S. H. Towards a molecular basis of neuronal recognition. In D. B. Tower (Ed.), *The nervous system. Vol. 1: The Basic Neurosciences.* New York: Raven, 1975.

Beach, F. A., & Jordan, L. Sexual exhaustion and recovery in the male rat. *Quarterly Journal of Experimental Psychology*, 1956, *8*, 121-133.

Beale, G. H. The antigen system of *Paramecium aurelia*. *International Review of Cytology*, 1957, *6*, 1-23.

Beránek, R., & Hník, P. Long term effects of tenotomy on spinal monosynaptic response in the cat. *Science*, 1959, *130*, 981-982.

Berg, D. K., & Hall, Z. W. Fate of alpha-bungarotoxin bound to acetylcholine receptors of normal and denervated muscle. *Science* (Washington, D.C.), 1974, *4*, 473-474.

Berger, T. W., Alger, B., & Thompson, R. F. Neuronal substrate of classical conditioning in the hippocampus. *Science*, 1976, *192*, 483-485.

Berlyne, D. E. *Conflict, arousal and curiosity.* New York: McGraw-Hill, 1960.

Berson, S. A., & Yalow, R. S. The present status of insulin antagonists in plasma. *Diabetes*, 1964, *13*, 247-259.

Berthelson, S., & Pettinger, W. A. A functional basis for classification of alpha-adrenergic receptors. *Life Sciences*, 1977, *21*, 595-606.

Beswick, F. B., & Conroy, R. T. W. L. Optimal tetanic conditioning of heteronymous monosynaptic reflexes. *Journal of Physiology* (London), 1965, *180*, 134-146.

Biederman, G. B., D'Amato, M. R., & Keller, D. M. Facilitation of discrimination avoidance learning by dissociation of CS and manipulandum. *Psychonomic Science*, 1964, *1*, 229-230.

Bitterman, M. E. Classical conditioning in the goldfish as a function of the CS-US interval. *Journal of Comparative and Physiological Psychology*, 1964, *58*, 359-366.

Bloom, F. E. Amine receptors in the CNS. I. Norepinephrine. In L. L. Iversen, S. D. Iversen, & S. H. Snyder (Eds.), *Handbook of psychopharmacology* (Vol. 6). New York: Plenum, 1975.

Bockaert, J., Roy, C., Rajerison, R., & Jard, S. Specific binding of (^{3}H)lysine-vasopressin to pig kidney membranes: Relationship of receptor occupancy to adenylate cyclase activation. *Journal of Biological Chemistry*, 1973, *248*, 5922-5931.

Bolles, R. C. Species-specific defense reactions and avoidance learning. *Psychological Review*, 1970, *77*, 32-48.

Bolles, R. C. Species-specific defense reactions. In F. R. Brush (Ed.), *Aversive conditioning and learning.* New York: Academic, 1971.

Bolles, R. C., Stokes, L. W., & Younger, M. S. Does CS termination reinforce avoidance behavior? *Journal of Comparative and Physiological Psychology*, 1966, *62*, 201-207.

Boyse, E. A., Old, L. J., & Leull, S. Antigenic properties of experimental leukemias. II. Immunological studies *in vivo* with C57BL/6 radiation-induced leukemias. *Journal of the National Cancer Institute*, 1963, *31*, 987-995.

Brown, E. M., Hauser, D., Troxler, F., & Aurbach, G. D. Beta-adrenergic receptor interactions: Characterization of iodohydroxybenzylpindolol as a specific ligand. *Journal of Biological Chemistry*, 1976, *251*, 1232-1238.

Brown, J. S. Factors affecting self-punitive locomotor behavior. In. B. A. Campbell & R. M. Church (Eds.), *Punishment and aversive behavior.* New York: Appleton-Century-Crofts, 1969.

Brown, L., Dearnaley, D. P., & Geffen, L. B. Noradrenaline storage and release in the decentralized spleen. *Proceedings of the Royal Society, Series B.*, 1967, *168*, 48-56.

Brown, M. C., & Ironton, R. The fate of motor axon sprouts in a partially denervated mouse muscle when regenerating nerve fibres return. *Journal of Physiology* (London), 1976, *263*, 181P-182P.

Brown, M. C., Jansen, J. K. S., & Van Essen, D. Polyneuronal innervation of skeletal muscles in new-born rats and its elimination during maturation. *Journal of Physiology* (London), 1976, *261*, 387–422.

Bryant, P. J., Bryant, S. V., & French, V. Biological regeneration and pattern formation. *Scientific American*, 1977, *193*, 66–81.

Bunney, B. S., Walters, J. R., Roth, R. H., & Aghajanian, G. K. Dopaminergic neurons: Effect of antipsychotic drugs and amphetamine on single cell activity. *Journal of Pharmacology and Experimental Therapeutics*, 1973, *185*, 560–571.

Burt, D. R., Creese, I., & Snyder, S. H. Antischizophrenic drugs: Chronic treatment elevates dopamine binding in brain. *Science*, 1977, *196*, 326–328.

Buser, P. Higher functions of the nervous system. *Annual Review of Physiology*, 1976, *38*, 217–245.

Butler, R. A. Discrimination learning by rhesus monkeys to visual-exploration motivation. *Journal of Comparative and Physiological Psychology*, 1953, *46*, 95–98.

Butler, R. A. The differential effect of visual and auditory incentives on the performance of monkeys. *American Journal of Psychology*, 1958, *71*, 591–593.

Butler, R. A., & Harlow, H. F. Persistence of visual exploration in monkeys. *Journal of Comparative and Physiological Psychology*, 1954, *47*, 258–263.

Cangiano, A. & Lutzemberger, L. Partial denervation affects both denervated and innervated fibers in the mammalian skeletal muscles. *Science*, 1977, *196*, 542–545.

Cannon, W. B., & Rosenblueth, A. *The supersensitivity of denervated structures*. New York: Macmillan, 1949.

Castellucci, V. F., Carew, T. J., & Kandel, E. R. Cellular analysis of long-term habituation of the gill-withdrawal reflex of *Aplysia californica*. *Science*, 1979, *202*, 1306–1308.

Changeux, J.-P. The cholinergic receptor protein from fish electric organ. In L. L. Iversen, S. D. Iversn, & S. H. Snyder (Eds.) *Handbook of psychopharmacology* (Vol. 6). New York: Plenum, 1975.

Changeux, J.-P, & Danchin, A. Selective stabilisation of developing synapses as a mechanism for the specification of neuronal networks. *Nature*, 1976, *264*, 705–712.

Chiel, H., Yehuda, S., & Wurtman, R. J. Development of tolerance in rats to the hypothermic effects of *d*-amphetamine and apomorphine. *Life Sciences*, 1974, *14*, 483–488.

Cohen, B., Matsuo, U., & Raphan, T. Quantitative analysis of the velocity characteristics of optokinetic nystagmus and optokinetic after-nystagmus. *Journal of Physiology* (London), 1977, *270*, 321–344.

Cohen, J. B., & Changeux, J.-P. The cholinergic receptor protein in its membrane environment. *Annual Review of Pharmacology*, 1975, *15*, 83–103.

Coleman, W. R., & Berger, L. H. Utility scaling of intracranial reinforcement duration. *Physiology & Behavior*, 1978, *21*, 485–490.

Cooper, J. R., Bloom, F. E., & Roth, R. H. *The biochemical basis of neuropharmacology*. New York: Oxford University Press, 1978.

Cooper, R. Recording changes in electrical properties in the brain: The EEG. In R. D. Myers (Ed.), *Methods in Psychobiology 1*. London: Academic, 1971.

Costall, B., & Naylor, R. S. Dissociation of stereotyped biting responses and orobucco-lingual dyskinesias. *European Journal of Pharmacology*, 1976, *36*, 423–429.

Costentin, J., Marçais, H., Protais, P., Baudry, M., DeLaBaume, S., Martres, M.-P. & Schwartz, J.-C. Rapid development of hypersensitivity of striatal dopamine receptors by alpha-methylparatyrosine and its prevention by protein synthesis inhibitors. *Life Sciences*, 1977, *21*, 307–314.

Costentin, J., Protais, P., & Schwartz, J.-C. Rapid and dissociated changes in sensitivities of different dopamine receptors in mouse brain. *Nature*, 1975, *257*, 405–407.

Courtney, K., & Roper, S. Sprouting of synapses after partial denervation of frog cardiac ganglion. *Nature*, 1976, *259*, 317–319.

Creese, I., Burt, D. R. & Snyder, S. H. Dopamine receptor binding enhancement accompanies lesion-induced behavioral supersensitivity. *Science*, 1977, *197*, 596–598.

Creutzfeldt, O. D., Kuhnt, U., & Benveneto, L. A. An intracellular analysis of visual cortical neurons to moving stimuli: Response in co-operative neuronal network. *Experimental Brain Research*, 1974, *21*, 251-274.

Curtis, D. R., & Ryall, R. W. The excitation of Renshaw cells by cholinomimetics. *Experimental Brain Research*, 1966, *2*, 49-65.

Deguchi, T., & Axelrod, J. Supersensitivity and subsensitivity of the beta-adrenergic receptor in pineal gland regulated by catecholamine transmitter. *Proceedings of the National Academy of Sciences*, 1973, *70*, 2411-2414.

Dember, W. N. The new look in motivation. *American Scientist*, 1965, *53*, 409-427.

Dember, W. N., & Earl, R. W. Analysis of exploratory, manipulatory and curiosity behaviors. *Psychological Review*, 1957, *64*, 91-96.

Dember, W. N., & Fowler, H. Spontaneous alternation behavior. *Psychological Bulletin*, 1958, *55*, 412-428.

DeMeyts, P., Bianco, A. R., & Roth, J. Site-site interactions among receptors: Characterization of the negative cooperativity. *Journal of Biological Chemistry*, 1976, *251*, 1877-1888.

DeMeyts, P., & Roth, J. Cooperativity in ligand binding: A new graphic analysis. *Biochemical and Biological Research Communications*, 1975, *66*, 1118-1126.

DeMeyts, P., Roth, J., Neville, D. M. Jr., Gavin, J. R. III, & Lesniak, M. A. Insulin interactions with its receptors: Experimental evidence for negative cooperativity. *Biochemical and Biophysical Research Communications*, 1973, *55*, 154-161.

Descarries, L., Watkins, K. C., & Lapierre, Y. Noradrenergic axon terminals in the cerebral cortex of rat. III. Topometric ultrastructural analysis. *Brain Research*, 1977, *133*, 197-222.

Dismukes, K. Two-faced neurones. *Nature*, 1977, *269*, 104-105.

Dismukes, K., & Daly, J. W. Altered resonsiveness of adenosine 3′,5′-monophosphate generating systems in brain slices from adult rats after neonatal treatment with 6-hydroxydopamine. *Experimental Neurology*, 1975, *49*, 150-160.

Dominic, J. A., & Moore, K. E. Supersensitivity to the central stimulant actions of adrenergic drugs following discontinuation of a chronic diet of alpha-methyltyrosine. *Psychopharmacologia*, 1969, *15*, 96-101.

Eccles, J. C. Postsynaptic inhibition in the central nervous system. In G. C. Quarton, T. Melnechuk, & F. O. Schmitt (Eds.), *The neurosciences*. New York: Rockefeller University Press, 1967.

Edds, M. V. Neuronal specificity in neurogenisis. In G. C. Quarton, T. Melnechuk, & F. O. Schmitt (Eds.), *The neurosciences*. New York: Rockefeller University Press, 1967.

Ehinger, B. Synaptic connections of the dopaminergic retinal neurons. *Advances in Biochemical Psychopharmacology*, 1977, *16*, 299-306.

Eldefrawi, M. E., & Eldefrawi, A. T. Cooperativities in the binding of acetylcholine to its receptor. *Biochemical pharmacology*, 1973, *22*, 3145-3130.

Eldefrawi, M. E., Eldefrawi, A. T., Seifert, S., & O'Brian, R. D. Properties of inbrol-solubilized acetylcholine receptor from *Torpedo electroplax*. *Archives of Biochemistry and Biophysics*, 1972, *150*, 210-218.

Emmelin, N. Action of acetylcholine on the responsiveness of effector cells. *Experientia*, 1964, *20*, 275. (a)

Emmelin, N. Influence of degenerating nerve fibers on the responsiveness of salivary gland cells. *Journal of Physiology* (London), 1964, *171*, 132-138. (b)

Enero, M. A., Langer, S. Z., Rothlin, R. P., & Stefano, F. J. E. Role of the alpha-adrenoceptor in regulating noradrenaline overflow by nerve stimulation. *British Journal of Pharmacology*, 1972, *44*, 672-688.

Estes, W. K. An experimental study of punishment. *Psychological Monographs*, 1944, *57*(Whole No. 263).

Ettenberg, A., & Milner, P. M. Effects of dopamine supersensitivity on lateral hypothalamic self-stimulation in rats. *Pharmacology, Biochemistry & Behavior*, 1977, *7*, 507-514.

Evarts, E. V. Unit activity in sleep and wakefulness. In G. C. Quarton, T. Melnechuk, & F. O. Schmitt (Eds.), *The neurosciences*. New York: Rockefeller University Press, 1967.

Fambrough, D. M. Acetylcholine receptors: Revised estimates of extrajunctional receptor density in denervated rat diaphragm. *Journal of General Physiology*, 1974, *64*, 468-472.

Fantino, E., Weigele, S., & Lancy, D. Aggressive display in the Siamese fighting fish (*Betta splendens*). *Learning & Motivation*, 1972, *3*, 457-468.

Feeney, D., Pittman, J., & Wagner, H. Lateral inhibition and attention: Comments on the neuropsychological theory of Walley and Weiden. *Psychological Review*, 1974, *81*, 536-539.

Feltz, D., & DeChamplain, J. Enhanced sensitivity of caudate neurones to microiontophetic injections of dopamine in 6-hydroxydopamine treated cats. *Brain Research*, 1972, *43*, 601-605.

Fiorentini, A., & Maffei, L. Instability of the eye in the dark and proprioception. *Nature*, 1977, *269*, 330-331.

Fowler, H., & Miller, N. E. Facilitation and inhibition of runway performance by hind- and forepaw shock of various intensities. *Journal of Comparative and Physiological Psychology*, 1963, *56*, 801-805.

Fox, J. L. Methods map brain functions chemically. *Chemical & Engineering News*, 1978, *56*, 20-22.

Frank, E., Jansen, J. K. S., Lømo, T., & Westgaard, R. H. The interaction between foreign and original motor nerves innervating the soleus muscle of rats. *Journal of Physiology* (London), 1975, *247*, 725-743.

Frazier, W. A., Boyd, L. F., & Bradshaw, R. A. Properties of the specific binding of ^{125}I-nerve growth factor in responsive peripheral neurons. *Journal of Biological Chemistry*, 1974, *249*, 5513-5519.

French, V., Bryant, P. J., & Bryant, S. V. Pattern regulation in epimorphic fields. *Science*, 1976, *193*, 964-981.

Freychet, P., Rosselin, G., Rancon, F., Foucereau, M., & Broer, Y. Interactions of insulin and glucagon with isolated rat liver cells. I. Binding of the hormone to specific receptors. *Hormonal and Metabolic Research*, 1974, *5*(Suppl.), 72-78.

Gianutsos, G., Drawbaugh, R. B., Hynes, M. D., & Lal, H. Behavioral evidence for dopaminergic supersensitivity after chronic haloperidol. *Life Sciences*, 1974, *14*, 887-898.

Gillin, J. C., Mendelson, W. B., Sitaram, N., & Wyatt, R. J. The neuropharmacology of sleep and wakefulness. *Annual Review of Pharmacology and Toxicology*, 1978, *18*, 563-579.

Ginsberg, B. H., Cohen, R. M., & Kahn, C. R. Insulin-induced dissociation of receptors into subunits: Possible molecular concomitant of negative cooperativity. *Diabetes*, 1976, *25*(Suppl. 1).

Girdner, J. B. An experimental analysis of the behavioral effects of a perceptual consequence unrelated to organic drive states. *American Psychologist*, 1953, *8*, 354-355.

Glanzer, M. Curiosity, exploratory drive, and stimulus satiation. *Psychological Bulletin*, 1958, *55*, 302-315.

Glass, L. Patterns of supernumerary limb regeneration. *Science*, 1977, *198*, 321-322.

Gnegy, M. E., Uzunov, P., & Costa, E. Regulation of the dopamine stimulation of striatal adenylate cyclase by an endogenous Ca^{++}-binding protein. *Proceedings of the National Academy of Sciences*, 1976, *73*, 3887-3890.

Gnegy, M., Uzunov, P., & Costa, E. Participation of an endogenous Ca^{++}-binding protein activator in the development of drug-induced supersensitivity of striatal dopamine receptors. *Journal of Pharmacology and Experimental Therapeutics*, 1977, *202*, 558-564.

Goldfarb, J., & Muller, R. U. Occurrence of heteronymous monosynaptic reflexes following tenotomy, *Brain Research*, 1971, *28*, 553-555.

Goldfine, I. D. Binding of insulin to thymocytes from suckling and hypophysectomized rats: Evidence for two mechanisms of regulating insulin sensitivity. *Endocrinology*, 1975, *97*, 948-954.

Granit, R., & Rutledge, L. T. Surplus excitation in reflex action of motoneurones as measured by recurrent inhibition. *Journal of Physiology* (London), 1960, *154*, 288-307.

Grant, G., Vale, W., & Guillemin, R. Characteristics of the pituitary binding sites for thyrotropin-releasing factor. *Endocrinology*, 1973, *92*, 1629–1633.

Grillner, S. Locomotion in vertebrates: Central mechanisms and reflex interaction. *Physiological Reviews*, 1975, *55*, 247–304.

Grinnell, A. D., Rheuben, M. B., & Letinsky, M. S. Mutual repression of synaptic efficacy by pairs of foreign nerves innervating from skeletal muscles. *Nature*, 1977 *265*, 368–370.

Gross, C. G., Rocha-Miranda, C. E., & Bender, D. B. Visual properties of neurons in inferotemporal cortex of the macaque. *Journal of Neurophysiology*, 1972, *35*, 96–111.

Grossman, S. P. The role of dopaminergic pathways in learning. *Proceedings of the International Union of Physiological Sciences*, Paris, 1977, *12*, 693.

Gulley, R. L., Wenthold, R. J., & Neises, G. R. Remodeling of neuronal membranes as an early response to deafferentation. *Journal of Cell Biology*, 1977, *75*, 837–850.

Guthrie, E. R. *The psychology of learning.* New York: Harper, 1935.

Halász, N., Hökfelt, T., Ljungdahl, Å., Johansson, O., & Goldstein, M. Dopamine neurons in the olfactory bulb. *Advances in Biochemical Psychopharmacology*, 1977, *16*, 169–177.

Harrison, L. C., Martin, F. I. R., & Melick, R. A. Correlation between insulin receptor binding in isolated fat cells and insulin sensitivity in obese human subjects. *Journal of Clinical Investigation*, 1976, *58*, 1435–1441.

Harwitz, H. M. B. Conditioned responses in rats reinforced by light. *British Journal of Animal Behaviour*, 1956, *4*, 31–33.

Hayward, J. N. Functional and morphological aspects of hypothalamic neurons. *Physiological Reviews*, 1977, *57*, 574–658.

Hebb, D. O. *The organization of behavior.* New York: Wiley, 1949.

Hebb, D. O. Drives and the C. N. S. (Conceptual Nervous System). *Psychological Review*, 1955, *62*, 243–254.

Hedqvist, P. Modulating effect of prostaglandin E_2 on noradrenaline release from isolate cat spleen. *Acta Physiologica Scandinavica*, 1969, *75*, 511–512.

Hernández-Peón, R., Scherrer, H., & Jouvet, M. Modification of electrical activity in the cochlear nucleus during "attention" in unanesthetized cats. *Science*, 1956, *123*, 331–332.

Hess, R., Negishi, K., & Creutzfeldt, O. The horizontal spread of intracortical inhibition in the visual cortex. *Experimental Brain Research*, 1975, *22*, 415–419.

Hill, W. F. Activity as an autonomous drive. *Journal of Comparative and Physiological Psychology*, 1956, *49*, 15–19.

Hiude, R. A. *Animal behavior. A synthesis of ethology and comparative psychology.* New York: McGraw-Hill, 1970.

Hodos, W. Motivational properties of long duration brain stimulation. *Journal of Comparative and Physiological Psychology*, 1965, *59*, 219–224.

Horn, G., & Wiesenfeld, Z. Attention in the cat: Electrophysiological and behavioral studies. *Experimental Brain Research*, 1974, *21*, 67–82.

Huang, M., & Daly, J. W. Adenosine-elicited accumulation of cyclic AMP in brain slices: Potentiation by agents which inhibit uptake. *Life Sciences*, 1974, *14*, 489–503.

Huang, M., Ho, A. K. S., & Daly, J. W. Accumulation of cyclic $3',5'$-monophosphate in rat cerebral cortical slices. Stimulatory effects of alpha and beta adrenergic agents after treatment with 6-hydroxydopamine, 2,3,5-trihydroxyphenethylamine and dehydroxytryptamine. *Molecular Pharmacology*, 1973, *9*, 711–717.

Hubel, D. H., & Wiesel, T. N. Receptive fields of single neurones in the cat's striate cortex. *Journal of Physiology* (London), 1959, *148*, 574–591.

Hubel, D. H., & Wiesel, T. N. Receptive fields, binocular interaction and functional architecture in the cat's visual cortex. *Journal of Physiology* (London), 1962, *160*, 106–154.

Hubel, D. H., & Wiesel, T. N. Shape and receptive fields of cells in striate cortex of very young, visually inexperienced kittens. *Journal of Neurophysiology*, 1963, *26*, 994–1002. (a)

Hubel, D. H., & Wiesel, T. N. Shape and arrangement of columns in cat's striate cortex. *Journal of Physiology* (London), 1963, *165*, 559–568. (b)

Hubel, D. H., & Wiesel, T. N. Receptive fields and functional architecture in two non-striate visual areas (18 and 19) of the cat. *Journal of Neurophysiology*, 1965, *28*, 229–289.

Hull, C. L. *Principles of behavior.* New York: Appleton-Century-Crofts, 1943.

Huttunen, M. O. General model for the molecular events in synapses during learning. *Perspectives in Biology and Medicine*, 1973, *17*, 103–108.

Hyttel, J. Long-term effects of teflutixol on the synthesis and endogenous levels of mouse brain catecholamines. *Journal of Neurochemistry*, 1975, *25*, 681–686.

Hyttel, J., & Nielsen, I. M. Changes in catecholamine concentrations and synthesis rate in mouse brain during the "supersensitivity" phase after treatment with neuroleptic drugs. *Journal of Neurochemistry*, 1976, *27*, 313–315.

Ince, L. P., Bracker, B. S., & Alba, A. Reflex conditioning in a spinal man. *Journal of Comparative and Physiological Psychology*, 1978, *92*, 796–802.

Inestrosa, N. C., Ramírez, B. U., & Fernandez, H. L. Effects of denervation and of axoplasmic transport blockage on the *in vitro* release of muscle endplate acetylcholinesterase. *Journal of Neurochemistry*, 1977, *28*, 941–945.

Iuvone, P. M., Galli, C. L., Garrison-Gund, C. K., & Neff, N. H. Light stimulates tyrosine hydroxylase activity and dopamine synthesis in retinal neurons. *Science*, 1979, *202*, 901–902.

Jacobs, B. L., Asher, R., & Dement, W. C. Electrophysiological and behavioral effects of electrical stimulation of the raphe nuclei in cats. *Physiology & Behavior*, 1973, *11*, 489–495.

Jard, S., Roy, C., Barth, T., Rajerison, R., & Bockaert, J. Antidinretic hormone-sensitive kidney adenylate cyclase. *Advances in Cyclic Nucleotide Research*, 1975, *5*, 31–52.

Jaynes, J. *The origin of consciousness in the breakdown of the biocameral mind.* Toronto: University of Toronto Press, 1976.

Jouvet, M. The role of monoamines and acetylcholine containing neurons in the regulation of the sleep-waking cycle. *Ergebnisse der Physiologie* 1972, *64*, 166–307.

Kahn, C. R. Membrane receptors for hormones and neurotransmitters. *Journal of Cell Biology*, 1976, *70*, 261–286.

Kalisker, A., Rutledge, C. O., & Perkins, J. P. Effect of nerve degeneration by 6-hydroxydopamine on catecholamine-stimulated adenosine 3',5'-monophosphate formation in rat cerebral cortex. *Molecular Pharmacology*, 1973, *9*, 619–629.

Kamin, L. J. The effects of termination of the CS and avoidance of the US on avoidance learning: An extension. *Canadian Journal of Psychology*, 1957, *11*, 48–56.

Kamin, L. J., & Brimer, C. J. The effects of intensity on conditioned and unconditioned stimuli on a conditioned emotional response. *Canadian Journal of Psychology*, 1963, *17*, 194–198.

Katsev. R. Extinguishing avoidance responses as a function of delayed warning signal termination. *Journal of Experimental Psychology*, 1967, *75*, 339–344.

Katz, B., & Thesleff, S. A study of the "desensitization" produced by acetylcholine at the motor end-plate. *Journal of Physiology* (London), 1957, *138*, 63–80.

Katz, R. J. Inhibition-mediating dopamine receptors and the control of intracranial reward. *Psychopharmacology*, 1979, *61*, 39–41.

Kebabian, J. W., Zatz, M., Romero, J. A., & Axelrod, J. Rapid changes in rat pineal beta-adrenergic receptors: Alterations in (^{3}H) alprenodol binding and adenylate cyclase. *Proceedings of the National Academy of Sciences*, 1975, *72*, 3735–3739.

Kendall, H. T., Wolfe, B. B., Sporn, J. R., Poulos, B. K., & Molinoff, P. B. Effects of 6-hydroxydopamine on the development of the beta-adrenergic receptor/adenylate cyclase system in rat cerebral cortex. *Journal of Pharmacology and Experimental Therapeutics*, 1977, *203*, 132–143.

Kiianmaa, K., & Fuxe, K. The effects of 5,7-dihydroxytryptamine-induced lesions of the ascending 5-hydroxytryptamine pathways on the sleep-wakefulness cycle. *Brain Research*, 1977, *131*, 287–301.

Kimble, D. P. Choice behavior in rats with hippocampal lesions. In R. L. Isaacson & K. H. Pribram (Eds.), *The hippocampus* (Vol. 2). New York: Plenum, 1975.

Kish, G. B. Learning when the onset of illumination is used as a reinforcing stimulus. *Journal of Comparative and Physiological Psychology*, 1955, *48*, 261-264.

Klee, W. A., & Streaty, R. A. Narcotic receptor sites in morphine-dependent rats. *Nature*, 1974, *248*, 61-63.

Klett, R. P., Fulpuis, B. W., Cooper, D., Smith, M., Reich, E., & Possani, L. D. The acetylcholine receptor. I. Purification and characterization of a macromolecule isolated from *Electrophorus electricus*. *Journal of Biological Chemistry*, 1973, *248*, 6841-6853.

Ko, P. K., Anderson, M. J., & Cohen, M. W. Denervated skeletal muscle fibers develop discrete patches of high acetylcholine receptor density. *Science*, 1977, *196*, 540-542.

Kobayashi, H., Hashiguchi, T., & Ushiyama, N. S. Postsynaptic modulation of excitatory process in sympathetic ganglia by cyclic AMP. *Nature*, 1978, *271*, 268-270.

Kohonen, T., Lehtiö, P., & Rovamo, J. Modelling of neural associative memory. *Annales Academiae Scientiarum Fennicae*, 1974, *167*, 1-18.

Kohonen, T., Lehtiö, P., Rovamo, J., Hyvärinen, J., Bry, K., & Vainio, L. A principle of neural associative memory. *Neuroscience*, 1977, *2*, 1065-1076.

Kolata, G. B. Hormone receptors: How are they regulated? *Science*, 1977, *196*, 747-748, 800.

Konorski, J. *Integrative activity of the brain*. Chicago: University of Chicago Press, 1967.

Kozak, W., & Westerman, R. Plastic changes of spinal monosynaptic responses from tenotomized muscles in cats. *Nature*, 1961, *189*, 753-755.

Kraly, F. S., Carty, W. J., & Smith, G. P. Effects of pregastric food stimuli on meal size and intermeal interval in the rat. *Physiology & Behavior*, 1978, *20*, 779-784.

Kravitz, E. A. Acetylcholine, gamma-aminobutyric acid and glutamic acid: Physiological and chemical studies related to their roles as neurotransmitters. In G. C. Quarton, T. Melnechuk, & F. O. Schmitt (Eds.), *The neurosciences*. New York: Rockefeller University Press, 1967.

Krueger, B. K., Forn, J., Walters, J. R., Roth, R. H., & Greengard, P. Stimulation by dopamine of adenosine 3',5'-monophosphate formation in rat caudate nucleus: Effect of lesions of the nigro-striatal pathway. *Molecular Pharmacology*, 1976, *12*, 639-648.

Kuffler, S. W. Discharge patterns and functional organization of mammalian retina. *Journal of Neurophysiology*, 1953, *16*, 37-68.

Kuffler, S. W., Dennis, M. J., & Harris, A. J. The development of chemosensitivity in extrasynaptic areas of the neuronal surface after denervation of parasympathetic ganglion cells in the heart of the frog. *Proceedings of the Royal Society, Series B.*, 1971, *177*, 555-563.

Lake, N., & Jordan, L. M. Failure to confirm cyclic AMP as second messenger from norepinephrine in rat cerebellum. *Science*, 1974, *183*, 663-664.

Lambert, D. H., Spannbauer, P. M., & Parsons, R. L. Desensitisation does not selectively alter sodium channels. *Nature*, 1977, *268*, 553-555.

Langer, S. Z. Denervation supersensitivity. In L. L. Iversen, S. D. Iversen, & S. H. Snyder (Eds.), *Handbook of psychopharmacology* (Vol. 2) New York: Plenum, 1975.

Langer, S. Z., & Dubocovich, M. L. Subsensitivity of presynaptic alpha-adrenoceptors after exposure to noradrenaline. *European Journal of Pharmacology*, 1977, *41*, 87-88.

Lassen, N. A., Ingvar, D. H., & Skinkφj, E. Brain function and blood flow. *Scientific American*, 1978, *239*, 50-59, 1978.

Laurberg, S., & Hjorth-Simonsen, A. Growing central axons deprived of normal target neurones by neonatal X-ray irradiation still terminate in a precisely laminated fashion. *Nature*, 1977, *269*, 158-160.

Lavoie, P.-A., Collier, B., & Tenenhouse, A. Comparison of alpha-bungarotoxin binding to skeletal muscles after inactivity or denervation. *Nature*, 1976, *260*, 349-350.

Lefkowitz, R. J., Mullikin, D., Wood, C. L., Gore, T. B., & Mukherjee, C. Regulation of prostaglandin receptors by prostaglandins and guanine nucleotides in frog erythrocytes. *Journal of Biological Chemistry*, 1977, *252*, 5295-5303.

Lesniak, M. A., & Roth, J. Regulation of receptor concentration by homologous hormone. *Journal of Cell Biology*, 1976, *251*, 3720-3729.

Lester, H. A. The response to acetylcholine. *Scientific American*, 1977, *236*, 106-118.

Leuba, C. Toward some integration of learning theories: The concept of optimal stimulation. *Psychological Report*, 1955, *1*, 27-33.

Libet, B. The role of SIF cells in ganglionic transmission. *Advances in Biochemical Psychopharmacology*, 1977, *16*, 541-546.

Lidbrink, P. The effect of lesions of ascending noradrenaline pathways on sleep and waking in the rat. *Brain Research*, 1974, *74*, 19-40.

Limbird, L. E., DeMeyts, P., & Lefkowitz, R. J. Beta-adrenergic receptors: Evidence for negative cooperativity. *Biochemical and Biophysical Research Communications*, 1975, *64*, 1160-1168.

Livingston, R. B. Brain circuitry relating to complex behavior. In G. C. Quarton, T. Melnechuk, & F. O. Schmitt (Eds.), *The neurosciences*, New York: Rockefeller University Press, 1967.

Llinás, R. The cerebral cortex. In D. B. Tower (Ed.), *The nervous system, Vol. 1: The Basic Neurosciences*. New York: Raven, 1975.

Lømo, T. Are there silent synapses? *Trends in Biological Sciences*, 1978, *3*, N9-N12.

Lømo, T., & Rosenthal, J. Control of ACh sensitivity by muscle activity in the rat. *Journal of Physiology* (London), 1972, *221*, 493-513.

Lopes da Silva, F. H., & Arnolds, D. E. A. T. Physiology of the hippocampus and related structures. *Annual Review of Physiology*, 1978, *40*, 185-216.

Mackintosh, N. J. *The psychology of animal learning*. London: Academic, 1974.

Magavanik, L., & Vyskočil, F. Desensitization at the motor endplate. In H. P. Rang (Ed.), *Drug receptors*. London: Macmillan, 1973.

Mantovani, P., Bartolini, A., & Pepeu, G. Interrelationships between depaminergic and cholinergic systems in the cerebral cortex. In E. Costa & G. L. Gesse (Eds.), *Advances in biochemical psychopharmacology* (Vol. 16). New York: Raven, 1977.

Mark, R. Are there silent synapses? *Trends in Biological Sciences*, 1978, *3*, N9-N12.

Martres, M.-P., Baudry, M., & Schwartz, J.-C. Subsensitivity of noradrenaline-stimulated cyclic AMP accumulation in brain slices of *d*-amphetamine treated mice. *Nature*, 1975, *255*, 731-733.

Mason, S. T., & Fibiger, H. C. Noradrenaline and partial reinforcement in rats. *Journal of Comparative and Physiological Psychology*, 1978, *92*, 1110-1118.

Matthysse, S. Dopamine and selective attention. *Advances in biochemical psychopharmacology*, 1977, *16*, 667-669.

Maugh, T. H. Hormone receptors: New clues to the cause of diabetes. *Science*, 1976, *193*, 220-222, 252.

Maximilian, A. V., Risberg, J., & Prohovniki, I. Changes in cerebral circulation during problem solving and verbal memory. *Proceedings of the Fifth Scandinavian Meeting on Physiology and Behavior*, Helsinki, 1977, 29.

McClelland, D. C., Atkinson, J. W., Clark, R. A., & Lowell, E. L. *The achievement motive*. New York: Appleton-Century-Crofts, 1953.

McEntee, W. J., & Mair, R. G. Memory impairment in Korsakoff's psychosis: A correlation with brain noradrenaline activity. *Science*, 1979, *202*, 905-908.

McGinty, D. J., & Harper, R. M. Dorsal raphe neurons: Depression of firing during sleep in cats. *Brain Research*, 1976, *101*, 569-575.

McLennan, H., & Miller, J. J. The hippocampal control of neuronal discharge in the septum of the rat. *Journal of Physiology* (London), 1974, *237*, 607-624.

McReynolds, P. A restricted conceptualization of human anxiety and motivation. *Psychological Report*, 1956, *2*, 293-312.

Melvin, K. B., & Anson, J. E. Facilitative effect of punishment on aggressive behavior in the Siamese fighting fish. *Psychonomic Science*, 1969, *14*, 89-90.

Menaker, M., Takahashi, J. S., & Eskin, A. The physiology of circadian pacemakers. *Annual Review of Physiology*, 1978, *40*, 501-526.

Mickey, J., Tate, R., & Lefkowitz, R. J. Subsensitivity of adenylate cyclase and decreased beta-adrenergic receptor binding after chronic exposure to (-)-isoproterenol *in vitro*. *Journal of Biological Chemistry*, 1975, *250*, 5727-5729.

Milner, P. M. The cell assembly: Mark II. *Psychological Review*, 1957, *64*, 242-252.

Misanin, J. R., Campbell, B. A., & Smith, N. F. Duration of punishment and the delay of punishment gradient. *Canadian Journal of Psychology*, 1966, *20*, 407-412.

Mishra, R. K., Gardner, E. L., Katzman, R., & Makman, M. H. Enhancement of dopamine-stimulated adenylate cyclase activity in rat caudate after lesions in substantia nigra: evidence for denervation supersensitivity. *Proceedings of the National Academy of Sciences*, 1974, *71*, 3883-3887.

Miyamoto, M. D., & Breckenridge, B. A cyclic adenosine monophosphate link in the catecholamine enhancement of transmitter release at the neuromuscular junction. *Journal of General Physiology*, 1974, *63*, 609-624.

Monnier, M., Dudler, L., Gaechter, R., Maier, P. F., Tobler, H. J., & Schoewenberger, G. A. The delta sleep inducing peptide (DSIP). Comparative properties of the original and synthetic nonapeptide. *Experientia*, 1977, *33*, 548-552.

Monod, J. *Chance and necessity*. New York: Vintage Books, 1972.

Moore, K. E., & Thornburg, J. E. Drug-induced dopaminergic supersensitivity. *Advances in Neurology*, 1975, *9*, 93-104.

Mora, F. The neurochemistry of brain self-stimulation. *Proceedings of the International Union of Physiological Sciences*, Paris, 1977, *12*, 687.

Morse, W. H., Mead, R. N., & Kelleher, R. T. Modulation of elicited behavior by a fixed-interval schedule of electric shock presentation. *Science*, 1967, *157*, 215-217.

Mountcastle, V. B. The problem of sensing and the neural coding of sensory events. In G. C. Quarton, T. Melnechuk, & F. O. Schmitt (Eds.), *The neurosciences*. New York: Rockefeller University Press, 1967.

Mowrer, O. H., & Lamoreaux, R. R. Avoidance conditioning and signal duration—a study of secondary motivation and reward. *Psychological Monographs*, 1942, *54*(5, Whole No. 247).

Mukherjee, C., Caron, M. C., Coverstone, M., & Lefkowitz, R. J. Identification of adenylate cyclase-coupled beta-adrenergic receptors in frog erythrocytes with (-)-(^{3}H)-alprenolol. *Journal of Biological Chemistry*, 1975, *250*, 4869-4876.

Mukherjee, C., Caron, M. C., & Lefkowitz, R. J. Catecholamine-induced subsensitivity of adenylate cyclase associated with loss of beta-adrenergic receptor binding sites. *Proceedings of the National Academy of Sciences*, 1975, *72*, 1945-1949.

Mukherjee, C., & Lefkowitz, R. J. Regulation of beta adrenergic receptors in isolated frog erythrocyte plasma membranes. *Molecular Pharmacology*, 1977, *13*, 291-303.

Muller, P., & Seeman, P. Brain neurotransmitter receptors after long-term haloperidol: Dopamine, acetylcholine, serotonin, alpha-noradrenergic and naloxone receptors. *Life Sciences*, 1977, *21*, 1751-1758.

Nagasaki, H., Iriki, M., & Uchizono, K. Inhibitory effect of the brain extract from sleep-deprived rats (BESDR) on the spontaneous discharges of crayfish abdominal ganglion. *Brain Research*, 1976, *109*, 202-205.

Nathanson, J. A. Cyclic nucleotides and nervous system function. *Physiological Reviews*, 1977, *57*, 157-256.

Nathanson, J. A., & Greengard, P. "Second messengers" in the brain. *Scientific American*, 1977, *237*, 108-119.

Natsoulas, T. Consciousness. *American Psychologist*, 1978, 33, 906-914.

Neher, E., & Sakmann, B. Single-channel currents recorded from membrane of denervated frog muscle fibres. *Nature*, 1976, *260*, 799-802.

Norman, J. L., Pettigrew, J. D., & Daniels, J. D. Early development of *X*-cells in kitten lateral geniculate nucleus. *Science*, 1977, *198*, 202-204.

Oldendorf, W. H. Permeability of the blood-brain barrier. In D. B. Tower (Ed.), *The nervous system, Vol. 1: The basic neurosciences.* New York: Raven, 1975.

Olds, J., & Olds, M. E. Drives, rewards and the brain. In T. M. Newcomb (Ed.), *New directions in psychology II.* New York: Holt, Rinehart & Winston, 1965.

Olefsky, J. M. The insulin receptor: Its role in insulin resistance and diabetes. *Diabetes,* 1976, *25,* 1154-1162.

Palmer, G. C. Increased cyclic AMP response to norepinephrine in the rat brain following 6-hydroxydopamine. *Neuropharmacology,* 1972, *11,* 145-149.

Palmer, G. C., Sulser, F., & Robinson, G. A. Effects of neurohumoral and adrenergic agents on cyclic AMP levels in various areas of the rat brain *in vitro. Neuropharmacology,* 1973, *12,* 327-337.

Pappenheimer, J. R., Koski, G., Fencl, V., Karnovsky, M. L., & Krueger, J. Extraction of sleep-promoting Factor S from cerebrospinal fluid and from brains of sleep-deprived animals. *Journal of Neurophysiology,* 1975, *38,* 1299-1311.

Patrick, J., Heinemann, S. F., Lindstrom, J., Schubert, D., & Steinbach, J. H. Appearance of acetylcholine receptors during differentiation of a myogenic cell line. *Proceedings of the National Academy of Sciences,* 1972, *69,* 2762-2766.

Pavlov, I. P. *Conditioned reflexes.* Oxford: Oxford University Press, 1927.

Pearson, K. The control of walking. *Scientific American,* 1976, *235,* 72-86.

Peckham, G. W., & Peckham, E. G. Some observations on the mental powers of spiders. *Journal of Morphology,* 1887, *1,* 383-419.

Perkins, J. P. Regulation of adenylate cyclase activity by neurotransmitters and its relation to neural function. In D. B. Tower (Ed.), *The nervous system, Vol. 1: The basic neurosciences.* New York: Raven, 1975.

Pert, C. B., Pasternak, G., & Snyder, S. H. Opiate agonists and antagonists discriminated by receptor binding in brain. *Science,* 1973, *182,* 1359-1361.

Pestronk, A., Drachman, D. B., & Griffin, J. W. Effect of muscle disuse on acetylcholine receptors. *Nature,* 1976, *260,* 352-353.

Pittman, J. C., & Feeney, D. M. Modulation of recurrent inhibition in cat association cortex by reticulocortical arousal. *Experimental Neurology,* 1974, *44,* 160-170.

Polak, R. L. Stimulating action of atropine on the release of acetylcholine by rat cerebral cortex *in vitro. British Journal of Pharmacology,* 1971, *41,* 600-606.

Premack, D. Reversibility of the reinforcement relation. *Science,* 1962, *136,* 255-257.

Premack, D., & Bahwell, R. Operant-level lever pressing by a monkey as a function of interest interval. *Journal of the Experimental Analysis of Behaviour,* 1959, *2,* 127-131.

Premack, D., Collier, G., & Roberts, C. L. Frequency of light-contingent bar pressing as a function of the amount of deprivation for light. *American Psychologist,* 1957, *12,* 411.

Premont, J., Tassin, J. P., Thierry, A. M., & Bockaert, J. Repartition and drug sensitivity of dopamine and L-isoproterenol-sensitive adenylate cyclase in rat brain homogenate. *Advances in Biochemical Psychopharmacology,* 1976, *15,* 347-356.

Purves, D. Competitive and non-competitive re-innervation of mammalian sympathetic neurons by native and foreign fibres. *Journal of Physiology* (London), 1976, *261,* 453-475.

Purves, D., & Sakmann, B. The effect of contractile activity on fibrillation and extrajunctional acetylcholine-sensitivity in rat muscle maintained in organ culture. *Journal of Physiology* (London), 1974, *237,* 157-182.

Raff, M. Self regulation of membrane receptors. *Nature,* 1976, *259,* 265-266.

Raisman, G. Evidence that new synaptic connections can be formed after injury to the central and peripheral nervous system in adult rats. *Acta Anatomica Nipponica,* 1977, *52,* 12-14.

Razran, G. The dominance-contiguity theory of the acquisition of classical conditioning. *Psychological Bulletin,* 1957, *54,* 1-46.

Reas, H. W., & Trendelenburg, U. Changes in the sensitivity of the sweat glands of the cat after denervation. *Journal of Pharmacology and Experimental Therapeutics,* 1967, *156,* 126-136.

Robbins, N., & Fischbach, G. Effect of chronic disuse of rat soleus neuromuscular junction on presynaptic function. *Journal of Neurophysiology*, 1971, *34*, 570–578.

Robbins, N., & Nelson, P. G. Tenotomy and the spinal monosynaptic reflex. *Experimental Neurology*, 1970, *27*, 66–75.

Roberts, C. L., Marx, M. H., & Collier, G. Light-onset and light-offset as reinforcers for the albino rat. *Journal of Comparative and Physiological Psychology*, 1958, *51*, 575–579.

Roberts, E. Disinhibition as an organizing principle in the nervous system—the role of gamma-aminobutyric acid. *Advances in Neurology*, 1974, *5*, 127–143.

Roberts, W. W. Both rewarding and punishing effects from stimulation of posterior hypothalamus of cat with same electrode at same intensity. *Journal of Comparative and Physiological Psychology*, 1958, *51*, 400–407.

Rochester, N., Holland, J. H., Haibt, L. H., & Duda, W. C. Tests of a cell assembly theory of the action of the brain using a large digital computer. *IRE Trans. Information Theory, IT.2, Symposium on Information Theory*, 1956, 80–93.

Rolls, E. T. *The brain and reward*. Oxford: Pergamon, 1975.

Roper, S. The acetylcholine sensitivity of the surface membrane of multiple-innervated parasympathetic ganglion cells in the mudpuppy before and after partial denervation. *Journal of Physiology (London)*, 1976, *254*, 455–473.

Roth, J., Neville, D. M., Kahn, C. R., & Gorden, D. Hormone resistance and hormone sensitivity. *New England Journal of Medicine*, 1977, *296*, 277–278.

Rowland, V. Steady potential phenomena of cortex. In G. C. Quarton, T. Melnechuk, & F. O. Schmitt (Eds.), *The neurosciences*. New York: Rockefeller University Press, 1967.

Royce, J. R. Psychology is multi-methodological, variate, epistemic, world-view, systemic, paradigmatic, theoretic, and disciplinary. In W. J. Arnold (Ed.), *Nebraska symposium on conceptual foundations of psychology*. Lincoln, Neb.: University of Nebraska Press, 1976.

Rubin, R. P. The role of calcium in the release of neurotransmitter substances and hormones. *Pharmacological Reviews*, 1970, *22*, 389–428.

Sandler, M., Ruthven, C. R. J., Goodwin, B. L., Reynolds, G. P., Rao, V. A. R., & Coppen, A. Deficient production of tyramine and octopamine in cases of depression. *Nature*, 1979, *278*, 357–388.

Sargent, P. B., & Dennis, M. J. Formation of synapses between parasympathetic neurons deprived of preganglionic innervation. *Nature*, 1977, *268*, 456–458.

Scheff, S., Benardo, L., & Cotman, C. Progressive brain damage accelerates sprouting in the adult rat. *Science*, 1977, *197*, 795–797.

Schmitt, F. O., Dev, P., & Smith, B. H. Electronic processing of information by brain cells. *Science*, 1976, *193*, 114–120.

Segal, M., & Olds, J. Activity of units in the hippocampal circuit of the rat during differential classical conditioning. *Journal of Comparative and Physiological Psychology*, 1973, *82*, 195–204.

Sharpless, S. K. Suprasensitivity-like phenomena in the central nervous system. *Federation Proceedings*, 1975, *34*, 1990–1997.

Shepherd, G. M. Microcircuits in the nervous system. *Scientific American*, 1978, *238*, 92–103.

Shinkman, P. G., & Bruce, C. J. Binocular differences in cortical receptive fields of kittens after rotationally disparate binocular experience. *Science*, 1977, *197*, 285–287.

Siggins, G. R., Hoffer, B. J., & Ungerstedt, U. Electrophysiological evidence for involvement of cyclic adenosine monophosphate in dopamine response of caudate nucleus. *Life Sciences*, 1974, *15*, 779–792.

Silverman, H. J., & Zucker, I. Absence of post-fast food compensation in the golden hamster (*Mesocricetus auratus*). *Physiology & Behavior*, 1976, *17*, 271–285.

Sinclair, J. D. The alcohol-deprivation effect in monkeys. *Psychonomic Science*, 1971, *25*, 21–22.

Sinclair, J. D. A theory of behavior based on "rest principle" control of the strength of neural connections. *Neuroscience & Biobehavioral Reviews*, 1978, *2*, 357–366.

Sinclair, J. D. Alcohol-deprivation effect in rats genetically selected for their ethanol preference. *Pharmacology, Biochemistry & Behavior*, 1979, *10*, 579–602.

Sinclair, J. D., & Bender, D. O. Compensatory behaviors: Suggestion for a common basis from deficits in hamsters. *Life Sciences*, 1978, *22*, 1407–1412.

Sinclair, J. D., & Senter, R. J. Increased preference for ethanol in rats following alcohol deprivation. *Psychonomic Science*, 1967, *8*, 11–12.

Sinclair, J. D., & Senter, R. J. Development of an alcohol-deprivation effect in rats. *Quarterly Journal of Studies on Alcohol*, 1968, *29*, 863–867.

Sinclair, J. D., & Sheaff, B. A negative alcohol-deprivation effect in hamsters. *Quarterly Journal of Studies on Alcohol*, 1973, *34*, 71–77.

Sinclair, J. D., Walker, S., & Jordan, W. Behavioral and physiological changes associated with various durations of alcohol deprivation. *Quarterly Journal of Studies on Alcohol*, 1973, *34*, 744–757.

Singer, W. The effect of mesencephalic reticular stimulation on intracellular potentials of cat lateral geniculate neurons. *Brain Research*, 1973, *61*, 35–54.

Singer, W. Control of thalamic transmission by corticofugal and ascending reticular pathways in the visual system. *Physiological Reviews*, 1977, *57*, 386–420.

Sloan, L. R., & Latane, B. Social deprivation and stimulus satiation in the albino rat. *Journal of Comparative and Physiological Psychology*, 1974, *87*, 1148–1156.

Smith, M. C., Coleman, S. R., & Gormezano, I. Classical conditioning of the rabbit's nictating membrane response at backward, simultaneous and forward CS–US intervals. *Journal of Comparative and Physiological Psychology*, 1969, *69* 226–231.

Soll, A. H., Kahn, C. R., & Neville, D. M. Jr. Insulin binding to liver plasma membranes in the obese hyperglycemic (ob/ob) mouse: Demonstration of a decreased number of functionally normal receptors. *Journal of Biological Chemistry*, 1975, *250*, 7402–7407.

Soll, A. H., Kahn, C. R., Neville, D. M. Jr., & Roth, J. Insulin receptor deficiency in genetic and acquired obesity. *Journal of Clinical Investigation*, 1975, *56*, 769–780.

Solomon, R. L., Kamin, L. J., & Wynne, L. C. Traumatic avoidance learning: The outcomes of several extinction procedures with dogs. *Journal of Abnormal and Social Psychology*, 1953, *48*, 291–302.

Soltysik, S. Inhibitory feedback in avoidance learning. *Boletín del Instituto de Estudios Médicos y Biológicos*, 1963, *21*, 433–449.

Spencer, W. A., & April, R. Plastic properties of monosynaptic pathways in mammals. In G. Horn & R. Hinde (Eds.), *Basic mechanisms of the epilepsies*. Boston: Little, Brown, 1969.

Spencer, W. A., & Kandel, E. R. Cellular and integrative properties of hippocampal pyramidal cell and the comparative electrophysiology of neurons. *International Journal of Neurology*, 1968, *6*, 266–296.

Spencer, W. A., & Wigdor, R. Ultra-late PTP monosynaptic reflex in cat. *Physiologist*, 1965, *8*, 278.

Sperling, G., & Melchner, M. J. The attention operating characteristic: Examples from visual search. *Science*, 1978, *202*, 315–318.

Spinelli, D. N., & Jensen, F. E. Plasticity: The mirror of experience. *Science*, 1979, *203*, 75–78.

Sporn, J. R., Harden, T. K., Wolfe, B. B., & Malinoff, P. B. Beta-adrenergic receptor involvement in 6-hydroxydopamine-induced supersensitivity in rat cerebral cortex. *Science*, 1976, *194*, 624–626.

Starke, K. Influence of extracellular noradrenaline on the stimulation-evoked secretion of noradrenaline from sympathetic nerves: Evidence for an alpha-receptor-mediated feed-back inhibition of noradrenaline release. *Naunyn-Schmiedebergs Archiv für Experimentelle Pathologie u. Pharmakologie*. 1972, *275*, 11–23.

Steinbach, J. H. Role of muscle activity in nerve-muscle interaction *in vitro*. *Nature*, 1974, *248*, 70–71.

Steriade, M. Cortical long-axoned cells and putative interneurons during the sleep-waking cycle. *The Behavioral and Brain Sciences*, 1978, *1*, 465-514.

Steriade, M., Deschenes, M., & Oakson, G. Inhibitory processes and interneuronal apparatus in motor cortex during sleep and waking. I. Background firing and responsiveness of pyramidal tract neurons and interneurons. *Journal of Neurophysiology*, 1974, *37*, 1065-1092.

Stjärne, L. Basic mechanisms and local feedback control of secretion of adrenergic and cholinergic neurotransmitters. In L. L. Iversen, S. D. Iversen, & S. H. Snyder (Eds.), *Handbook of psychopharmacology* (Vol. 6). New York: Plenum, 1975.

Stjärne, L., & Brundin, J. β_2-adrenoceptors facilitating noradrenaline secretion from human vasoconstrictor muscles. *Acta Physiologica Scandinavica*, 1976, *97*, 88-93.

Stjärne, L., & Brundin, J. Prostaglandin E_2- and alpha- or beta-adrenoceptic mediated interferences with ^{3}H-noradrenaline secretion from human vasomotor nerve: Comparison between effects on omental arteries and veins. *Acta Physiologica Scandinavica*, 1977, *100*, 267-269. (a)

Stjärne, L., & Brundin, J. Frequency-dependence of ^{3}H-noradrenaline secretion from human vasoconstrictor nerves: Modification by factors interfering with alpha- or beta-adrenoceptor or prostaglandin E_2 mediated control. *Acta Physiologica Scandinavica*, 1977, *101*, 199-210. (b)

Strada, S. J., Uzunov, P., & Weiss, B. Increased sensitivity to norepinephrine of the cyclic 3',5'-adenosine monophosphate system of rat brain following 6-hydroxydopamine. *Pharmacologist*, 1971, *13*, 257.

Sytkowski, A. J., Vogel, Z., & Nirenberg, M. W. Development of acetylcholine receptor clusters on cultured muscle cells. *Proceedings of the National Academy of Sciences*, 1973, *70*, 270-274.

Tarsy, D., & Baldessarini, R. J. Behavioral supersensitivity to apomorphine following treatment with drugs which interfere with the synaptic function of catecholamines. *Neuropharmacology*, 1974, *13*, 927-940.

Tate, R. L., Holmes, J. M., Kohn, L. D., & Winard, R. Characteristics of a solubilized thyrotropin receptor from bovine thyroid plasma membrane. *Journal of Biological Chemistry*, 1975, *250*, 6527-6535.

Thompson, R. F. & Spenser, W. A. Habituation: A model for the study of neuronal substrates of behavior. *Psychological Review*, 1966, *173*, 16-43.

Toates, F. M. Homeostasis and drinking. *The Behavioral and Brain Sciences*, 1979, 2, 95-102.

Treisman, A. Strategies and models of selective attention. *Psychological Review*, 1969, *76*, 282-299.

Trendelenburg, U. Supersensitivity and subsensitivity to sympathomimetic amines. *Pharmacological Reviews*, 1963, *15*, 225-276.

Trendelenburg, U., Maxwell, R. A., & Pluchino, S. Methoxamine as a tool to assess the importance of intraneuronal uptake of L-norepinephrine in the cat's nictating membrane. *Journal of Pharmacology and Experimental Therapeutics*, 1970, *172*, 91-99.

Trulson, M. M., & Jacobs, B. L. Behavioral evidence for denervation supersensitivity after destruction of central serotonergic nerve terminals. *Annals of the New York Academy of Sciences*, 1978, *305*, 497-509.

Tsumoto, T., & Suzuki, D. A. Effects of frontal eye field stimulation upon activities of the lateral geniculate body of the cat. *Experimental Brain Research*, 1976, *25*, 291-306.

Turner, L. H., & Solomon, R. L. Human traumatic avoidance learning: Theory and experiments on the operant-respondent distinction and failure to learn. *Psychological Monographs*, 1962, 76(40, Whole No. 559).

Ungerstedt, U. Striatal dopamine release after amphetamine or nerve degeneration revealed by rotational behavior. *Acta Physiologica Scandinavica*, 1971, *367*, 49-68. (a)

Ungerstedt, U. Postsynaptic supersensitivity after 6-hydroxydopamine induced degeneration of the nigro-striatal dopamine system. *Acta Physiologica Scandinavica, Supplement*, 1971, *367*, 69-93 (b)

Van Essen, D., & Jansen, J. K. Reinnervation of the rat diaphragm during perfusion with alpha-bungarotoxin. *Acta Physiologica Scandinavica*, 1974, *91*, 571-573.

Verrier, B., Fayet, G., & Lisitzky, S. Thyrotropin-binding properties of isolated thyroid cells and their purified plasma membranes. *European Journal of Biochemistry*, 1974, *42*, 355-365.

Vetulani, J., Stawarz, R. J., & Sulser, F. Adaptive mechanism of the noradrenergic cyclic AMP generating system in the limbic forebrain of the rat: Adaptation to persistant changes in the availability of norepinephrine. *Journal of Neurochemistry*, 1976, *27*, 661-666.

Vinogradova, O. S. Functional organization of the limbic system in the process of registration of information: Facts and hypotheses. In R. L. Isaacson & K. H. Pribram (Eds.), *The hippocampus* (Vol. 2). New York: Plenum, 1975.

Von Voigtlander, P. F., Boukma, S. J., & Johnson, G. A. Dopaminergic denervation supersensitivity and dopamine stimulated adenyl cyclase activity. *Neuropharmacology*, 1973, *12*, 1081-1086.

Von Voigtlander, P. F., Losey, E. G., & Triezenberg, H. J. Increased sensitivity to dopaminergic agents after chronic neuroleptic treatment. *Journal of Pharmacology and Experimental Therapeutics*, 1975, *193*, 88-94.

Waddington, J. L., & Cross, A. J. Denervation supersensitivity in the striatonigral GABA pathway. *Nature*, 1978, *276*, 618-620.

Wagner, A. R., Siegel, S., Thomas, E., & Ellison, G. D. Rineforcement history and the extinction of a conditioned salivary response. *Journal of Comparative and Physiological Psychology*, 1964, *58*, 354-358.

Walley, R. E., & Weiden, T. D. Lateral inhibition and cognitive masking. A neuropsychological theory of attention. *Psychological Review*, 1973, *80*, 284-302.

Walters, G. C., & Glazer, R. D. Punishment of instinctive behavior in the Mongolian gerbil. *Journal of Comparative and Physiological Psychology*, 1971, *75*, 331-340.

Wayner, M. J., Greenberg, R., Tartaglione, D. Nolley, S., Fraley, S., & Cott, A. A new factor affecting the consumption of ethyl alcohol and other sapid fluids. *Physiology & Behavior*, 1972, *8*, 345-362.

Wennmalm, Å. Quantitative evaluation of release and reuptake of adrenergic transmitter in the rabbit heart. *Acta Physiologica Scandinavica*, 1971, *82*, 532-538.

White, N., Brown, Z., & Yachnin, M. Effects of catecholamine manipulations on three different self-stimulation behaviors. *Pharmacology, Biochemistry & Behavior*, 1978, *9*, 273-278.

Williams, B. J., & Pirch, J. H. Correlation between brain adenyl cyclase activity and spontaneous motor activity in rats after chronic reserpine treatment. *Brain Research*, 1974, *68*, 227-234.

Wilson, D. F. The effects of dibutyryl cyclic adenosine 3′,5′-monophosphate, theophylline and aminophylline on neuromuscular transmission in the rat. *Journal of Pharmacology and Experimental Therapeutics*, 1974, *188*, 447-452.

Wirz-Justice, A., Krauchi, K., Lichtsteiner, M., & Feer, H. Is it possible to modify serotonin receptor sensitivity? *Life Sciences*, 1978, *23*, 1249-1254.

Woods, S. C., & McKay, L. D. Intraventricular alloxan eliminates feeding elicited by 2-deoxyglucose. *Science*, 1979, *202*, 1209-1210.

Wundt, W. *Grundzüge der physiologischen Psychologie*. Leipzig: Engelmann, 1874.

Yin, T. C. T., & Mountcastle, V. B. Visual input to the visuomotor mechanisms of the monkey's parietal lobe. *Science*, 1977, *197*, 1381-1383.

Yip, J. W., & Dennis, M. J. Suppression of transmission at foreign synapses in adult newt muscle involves reduction in quantal content. *Nature*, 1976, *260*, 350-352.

York, D. H. Possible dopaminergic pathway from substantia nigra to putamen. *Brain Research*, 1970, *20*, 233-241.

Young, D. N., Ellison, G. D., & Feeney, D. M. Electrophysiological correlates of selective attention: Modality specific changes in thalamo-cortical evoked potentials. *Brain Research*, 1971, *28*, 501-510.

Glossary of Abbreviations and Technical and Idiosyncratic Terms

Acetylcholine ($C_7H_{17}O_3N$): A transmitter substance released by neurons at most neuromuscular junctions and also at some synapses.

Action potential: The all-or-none spike generated by neurons, usually when the cumulative excitation exceeds a threshold value.

Additional assumption: That connections very slowly become weaker over long periods of inactivity, independent of changes caused by the *rest principle*.

Agonist: A chemical that fills a particular type of receptor, causing it to trigger the related cellular response.

Alpha-adrenergic receptors: Both alpha- and beta-adrenergic receptors bind norepinephrine, but some other agonists will bind to only one or the other type of receptor. Alpha-adrenergic receptors are generally on the presynaptic neuron and trigger a suppression of norepinephrine release, whereas beta-adrenergic receptors are generally postsynapatic or located on more distant target cells.

Antagonist: A substance that prevents a particular type of agonist and receptor from triggering their related cellular response.

Apomorphine: A dopaminergic agonist.

Antigenic modulation: The loss of surface antigens (like *receptors*) caused by the presence of many antibodies and the gain in antigens when the antibodies are gone.

Attention: (1) The general state of high awareness and receptivity; (2) the process that alters various mental abilities so that stimuli are perceived, thoughts pursued, or responses made, with less chance of disruption.

ATP (adenosine triphosphate): The immediate source of energy within cells for many functions.

Autonomous control of eating: Changes in the probability that eating will occur caused by *rest principle* alterations in the strength of the connections in the neural pathway producing the response, weakening the connections while the response is being made and strengthening them when the pathways are resting, as opposed to changes caused by homeostatic stimuli, other types of stimuli, and competing responses.

Aversion, conditioned taste: The decrease in the probability that a flavored substance will be consumed as a result of its previous consumption having been followed by nausea.

Backward conditioning: The classical conditioning paradigm in which the onset of the UCS precedes the onset of the CS.

Beta-adrenergic receptors: See *alpha-adrenergic receptors*.

Basket cells: Moderately large inhibitory interneurons found in the newer brain areas.

Blocking agent; blocker: An antagonist that acts by binding to the receptor in a way that does not trigger the cellular response but prevents agonists from binding.

cAMP (cyclic AMP; cyclic $3',5'$-adenosine monophosphate):   A chemical compound implicated in a wide variety of cellular functions, possibly including acting as a "second messenger" within the postsynaptic neuron.

Catecholamines: A group of hormones, transmitters, and modulators including norepinephrine, dopamine, and epinephrine.

Cerebellum: A newer brain structure with a highly ordered cytological architecture, important in motor functions (see Fig. 9.3).

Compensatory behaviors: Responses that become more likely to be emitted after a period in which they have not been made.

Concept neurons: Neurons excited by any of a general class of related stimuli (e.g., by the sight of any line with a particular orientation, of any apple, etc.).

Connection, neural: The set of all synapses from one neuron directly onto another.

Consumatory response: A general term for all actions in which substances are consumed (e.g., eating and drinking).

CS (conditioned stimulus):   A stimulus (e.g., the sound of a bell) that evokes a certain response (e.g., salivation) only after it has been paired with an unconditioned stimulus (e.g., food) that already evokes the response.

CS–UCS interval: The time duration between the onset of the conditioned stimulus and the onset of the unconditioned stimulus.

Cytological architecture: The anatomical pattern of neurons and their synapses within a structure.

Dendrodendritic synapse: A synapse from the dendrite of one neuron onto the dendrite of another neuron, as opposed to the classical synapse from an axon onto a dendrite (see Fig. 9.4).

Denervation supersensitivity: The reduced threshold or increased responsiveness of muscles, glands, and neurons to a transmitter, that develops after the nerve innervating the structure and releasing this transmitter has been cut.

Deprivation effect: The increased consumption of a substance to which one is accustomed, occurring immediately after a period when it is not available.

Discriminative stimulus: A signal that announces when a response will be followed by reinforcement.

Disuse supersensitivity: Like *denervation supersensitivity*, but caused by anything that prevents the transmitter from going to the receptors on the target structure.

DA (dopamine):   A transmitter and/or modulator between neurons.

Dopamine junction: A particular arrangement of neurons and synapses, including a small dopamine-releasing neuron, present at least in peripheral ganglia, that interact so that input to the junction makes it easier for subsequent input (up to 3 hours later) to produce output.

EEG (electroencephalograph):   Device for measuring the pattern of general electrical potentials ("brain waves") in areas of the brain.

EPSP (excitatory postsynaptic potential):   See *IPSP*.

Endorphine: A compound found normally in the body that fits the same receptors as morphine and other opiates, and probably acts as a transmitter and/or modulator.

Evoked potential: Stereotyped electrical changes, usually in cortical areas, produced by and occurring immediately after a stimulus.

Feature analyzer: A neuron that is excited only by a specific complex stimulus, or a specific component of the stimulus, and the neuronal network responsible for this behavior.

GABA (gamma aminobutyric acid):   An inhibitory transmitter substance, very common in the brain.

Golgi type II neurons: Small neurons found in all layers of the cerebral cortex (and elsewhere), probably acting with only graded potentials.

Graded potentials: Electrical changes in membranes that can be of any magnitude depending on the amount of stimulation, as opposed to action potentials that are all-or-none and of a magnitude (amplitude) independent of the input.

Granule cells: (1) In olfactory bulb, small inhibitory interneurons acting by graded potentials only; (2) in the hippocampus, excitatory neurons receiving input and giving output to the pyramidal cells. The term is used in this book also for stellate cells in the cerebral cortex that are believed to function similarly to the hippocampal granule cells.

Habituation: The weakening and eventual elimination of a response caused by the rapid repeated elicitation of the response.

Haloperidol: A dopaminergic blocking agent.

Hippocampus: A brain structure, relatively modern but more primitive than the cerebral cortex to which it is closely related (see Fig. 9.3).

Hypothalamus: An area at the base of the brain, characterized by the lack of a blood–brain barrier in some places and functioning to regulate substances in the blood (see Fig. 9.3).

ICSS (intracranial self-stimulation): Working in order to elicit electrical (or chemical) excitation of areas within the brain.

Interneuron: A neuron lying completely within a structure; more specifically, small neurons lying between the parallel pathways of the large neurons.

IPSP (inhibitory postsynaptic potential): The electrical changes in the membrane of a postsynaptic neuron caused by inhibitory transmitters that make it more difficult for excitatory postsynaptic potentials (EPSPs) to fire the neuron.

Korsakoff's syndrome: A particular combination of symptoms found together in some alcoholics, including the inability to remember recent events.

LGN (lateral geniculate nucleus): A portion of the thalamus relaying visual input (see Fig. 9.3).

Line detectors: Neurons excited by visual stimuli consisting of lines or straight edges between contrasting areas with a particular orientation.

Massed trials: Rapidly repeated trials.

Mnemonic system: A special procedure for improving the ability to memorize.

Modulator: A substance released by neurons that changes the activity of other neurons by means other than excitation or inhibition.

MRF (mesencephalic reticular formation): A portion of the midbrain implicated in the control of sleep and arousal.

NE (norepinephrine; noradrenaline): A neural transmitter and/or modulator.

Parkinson's disease: A syndrome characterized by rhythmic tremor and difficulty in making slow, smooth movements, treatable with L-dopa (a precursor of dopamine).

Posttetanic potentiation: The increased ease with which some neural pathways are traversed as a result of prior repetitive firing at a very rapid rate.

Priming: Increasing the probability or vigor of a learned response by giving a small amount of the positive reinforcement before the first response is made.

Pyramidal neurons: The generally large neurons of the hippocampus and cerebral cortex, usually responsible for output to other structures.

Receptor: A structure with a shape and/or electrical charges such that only substances with complementary shapes and/or charges are able to bind to it; the binding usually causes some change in the receptor and triggers a particular cellular response.

Response chain: A frequently used sequence of responses, usually occurring in a relatively fixed order and contributing to a common goal.

Rest principle: The strength of a neural connection becomes weaker if it is used repeatedly without rest but becomes stronger while the connection rests after use, with the largest increments occurring early in the rest period.

Reticular formation: A primitive portion of the nervous system, characterized by a lack of an ordered cytological architecture (see Fig. 9.3).

Serotonin (5HT, 5-hydroxytryptamine; $C_{10}H_{12}N_2O$):   A neural transmitter.

SIF cells (small intensely florescent cells):   The dopamine-releasing neurons found in the dopamine junctions of the sympathetic ganglia.

Silent synapse: A synapse in which the presynaptic neuron no longer releases enough transmitter under normal conditions to elicit a measurable electrical response in the postsynaptic neuron.

Simultaneous conditioning: The classical conditioning paradigm in which the UCS and CS begin at the same time.

Spontaneous alternation: The tendency of most animals to choose the opposite arm of a T-maze on the second trial to the one chosen on the first trial.

Stabilized retinal images: Stimuli projected onto the retina of the eye in such a way as to counteract eye movements, thus maintaining an unchanging level of illumination on each retinal cell.

Strength of a neural connection: The probability that a fixed amount of activity in the presynaptic neuron will be able to alter the activity of the postsynaptic neuron by a fixed amount via the direct synapses between them.

Terminator: The particular combination of stimuli that acts to stop a response chain.

Topological mapping: The similarity of spatial relations between points on the cortex and the points on the retina (or on the surface of the body) that excite the cortical points, such that a map of the retina (or body surface) is represented on the cortex.

Use principle: The strength of a neural connection becomes stronger the more the connection is used.

UCS (unconditioned stimulus):   The stimulus that already elicits the measured response, the UCR, before classical conditioning is performed.

6-Hydroxydopamine: A compound used to destroy neurons releasing catecholamines.

Author Index

Numbers in italic indicate the page on which the complete reference appears.

Subject Index

Page numbers in italics refer to figures and tables.

For Product Safety Concerns and Information please contact our EU
representative GPSR@taylorandfrancis.com Taylor & Francis Verlag GmbH,
Kaufingerstraße 24, 80331 München, Germany

Printed and bound by CPI Group (UK) Ltd, Croydon, CR0 4YY

01/05/2025

01858538-0001